Sex

and the

Bible

Sex
and the
Bible

Gerald Larue

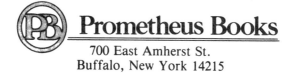

Prometheus Books
700 East Amherst St.
Buffalo, New York 14215

Published in 1983 by
Prometheus Books
700 East Amherst Street
Buffalo, New York 14215

Printed in the United States of America

Library of Congress Card Catalog No. 83-60201
ISBN: 0-87975-213-0

For Amber
a precious jewel
who has encouraged and sustained me

Contents

Preface

This book has developed out of a variety of educational and social experiences. For more than twenty years I taught courses in biblical history, literature, and archaeology at the University of Southern California. Scarcely a semester passed in which students did not raise questions about some of the attitudes toward sex found in the Bible. Some wrote term papers exploring what biblical writers said and the effect of their ancient ideas on modern life.

After I wrote *Ancient Myth and Modern Man* (1975), in which I commented on some of the biblical ideas about sex, I was invited each semester to give a lecture on the theme of ''The Bible and Human Sexuality'' in a human sexuality class taught by Dr. Laura Schlessinger. Student responses in this setting made it obvious that many, despite their religious background, had little understanding of what was in the Bible, but most had been profoundly touched or affected by the teachings of their synagogue or church. After-class conferences made me aware of the guilt many young people were carrying because they believed they had violated some divine precept set forth in the Bible.

About this same time I began to teach a class about death and dying, which also developed out of the *Ancient Myth and Modern Man* volume. The trauma associated with the fear of loss and separation, and the inner pain produced by death, became apparent immediately. To deal adequately with these emotional responses, I took some courses offered by the Department of Sociology at the university through the Human Relations Center and began to work toward certification as a marriage, family, and child counselor. The courses at the Center and my counseling experience both there and at the Out-patient Center of the Chabad Rehabilitation and Mental Health Programs, and most recently with the Taylor Therapy Center in Beverly Hills, acquainted me with new and helpful therapy for those whose responses and feelings have been affected—directly and indirectly—by what they believe the Bible or their religious affiliation teaches about acceptable sexual behavior.

Most recently, as Leader of the Ethical Culture Society of Los Angeles, I have had the rare privilege of being a participant on a radio program titled ''Religion on the Line'' (KABC, Los Angeles), moderated until recently by a beautiful and dynamic woman named Carol Hemingway. Many of the questions phoned in and fielded by the panel, which included a Roman Catholic priest, a rabbi, a Protestant minister, and myself, were concerned with the Bible and human sexuality. The responses of these compassionate religious leaders always focused on some facet of biblical teaching or their denominational interpretation of specific passages from the Bible.

At present, since I retired as Emeritus Professor of Religion from the University of Southern California, I have been teaching courses in ethics and values in aging at the Andrus Gerontology Center at the University of Southern California. Through the students and my colleagues, I am in touch with the way belief systems affect older citizens and their sexuality.

Clearly, there are many who have contributed to this book both directly and indirectly. They include students, friends, colleagues, and those anonymous individuals who shared their pain, confusion, and convictions by telephone and over the radio. To a select group I owe special thanks: to the instructors at the Human Relations Center, including Dr. Carlfred B. Broderick, Professor Marcia Laswell, Dr. Larry Altman, Dr. John Grenner, Dr. Richard Varnes, and Dr. Alexander Taylor. I owe much to Dr. Taylor, who invited me to join his staff at the Taylor Therapy Center as an intern therapist, and to Dr. Marion Schulman of the Taylor Therapy Center, who has been my supervisor. I am grateful to Edwin S. Cox, director of the California Family Study Center in Burbank, California, for the opportunity to teach a short course called "Religion and Therapy." Arthur L. de Munitiz provided me with references for various encyclopedias. From a friend and colleague of many years, Dr. Herman Harvey, a psychologist to whom I turn in time of stress or crisis (as I do to my two sons Dr. Gerald A. Larue, Jr., and Dr. David Larue), I have received much wise counsel. None of those I have mentioned have read this book and hence cannot be held responsible for any of the opinions I expressed.

Finally, I owe a great debt to Amber (Emily/Paula) Perkins, who in the last desperate moments of the completion of the manuscript typed into the late hours of the night to help me meet an already postponed deadline.

I also want to thank Paul Kurtz, the founder of Prometheus Books and a significant personal friend, for encouraging me to write this book. Doris Doyle, my editor at Prometheus, has been helpful, cooperative, and patient—three virtues that made our work together pleasant and productive.

Introduction

There is far more sex talk in the Bible than most people realize, and in one way or another what the Bible "says" about sex and human sexuality has a strong influence on our Western culture. No other ancient document affects our individual and group lives with the direct and subtle force of the Bible. Those who do not accept the Bible as an authoritative guide for faith and conduct are nevertheless touched in one way or another by what the clergy and members of synagogues and churches believe about it. How can that be?

Every day and every hour of the day, someone in some part of the Western world is studying the Bible, reading its chapters and verses for insight into the meaning and purpose of life, for the solution to personal problems, or for some indication of the shape of things to come from its prophetic writings. During every hour of every day the electronic media bring the interpretations of the Scriptures into hundreds and thousands and even millions of homes. Amid the constant pleas for money to support these radio and television ministers and their causes are exposition of verses and chapters of the Bible, exhortations to accept particular interpretations of certain portions of the writings, and a continuing insistence that the deity has provided the Bible as a guidebook to salvation. Whether one likes it or not the influence of the Bible is there—a reality. Whether or not one listens to radio and television preachers does not really matter either. Nor does it matter if one ever looks into a Bible. The influence is there.

We live in communities, and within each community there are those who hear and believe and attempt to obey what the Bible teaches. Some are content to apply their interpretations of the Bible to their own lives, others would "win the world for Christ." Such people interpret everything from the development of the state of Israel to whatever moves the Russians might make as some sort of fulfillment of biblical prophecy. They write letters to the newspapers and to influential government leaders. They belong to parent-teacher groups in local schools. They vote and work for their favorite candidates. They are in business. They are part of the local environment, and they make their presence felt within that environment. Thus, when some overzealous congressperson proposes legislation to prevent homosexuals from teaching in public schools and supports the position by quotations from the Bible, and when a popular singer gets on an anti-homosexual bandwagon, these same neighbors give support to these causes and turn their righteous anger or indignation or sense of outrage against local homosexuals. In other words, our lives are touched by the Bible by the very fact that we live in a nation where many people believe (or think they believe) in the authority of the Bible and are willing to back that belief openly, vociferously, and with the contribution of money.

During the many different religious festivals, merchants capitalize on them by selling special merchandise. The biggest religio-commercial enterprise is Christmas, but Passover, Easter, and other times of religious celebration are also advertised and merchandised. One would have to be completely isolated not to be influenced either positively or negatively by these public statements about religion.

None of these influences are directly linked to human sexuality, except perhaps the legislation pertaining to homosexual rights; but the idea that the Bible is to be looked to for guidance is taught indirectly. The Bible's influence on attitudes toward human sexuality is more subtle. Through churches and synagogues, and through parents and grandparents and other relatives, through neighbors and members of peer groups, all of whom may have had some education in religious thinking, the attitudes of growing children are shaped. Children may or may not be told directly that God does not approve of certain kinds of sexual thinking, talking, and acting, but in one way or another they will feel and respond to the life-shaping influence of these ideas.

As infants, as we begin to explore our bodies, we are told by parents and others that certain areas are "no-no" or "no touch" regions. As we mature, the adult world continues to shape us. Our parents were affected by what their parents believed, and through the ages this familial leavening has gone on, subtly transmitted through environmental and relational conditioning. Throughout this long period, the Bible and biblical taboos have played their part.

In the beginning, children are made to feel guilt when they violate parental wishes and standards. They are taught that they "ought" to feel unhappy because they have been told that when they "fail" to be "good children" they "disappoint" their parents. As they grow a bit older, the church and the synagogue assume parental roles and teach young people about God's will and God's rules and regulations as set forth in various parts of the Bible. They are told what is "natural" and "normal" and "good" and warned against what is "unnatural," "abnormal," and "evil." As they violate these standards, the weight of guilt is increased.

Added to familial and religious teachings are the bits of folkloric information that are always in circulation and seem to come into the consciousness of youth by some sort of communal osmosis but which are in reality passed on by peers who learn this folk wisdom from relatives—aunts, uncles, grandparents—with some contribution from neighbors. If these parental, religious, and folkloric notions are not challenged and, if necessary, countered by evidence, they remain uncorrected and can affect sexual behavior, generating all sorts of fears and doubts. For example, it was said that masturbation could drive a person insane; that each drop of semen ejaculated during a masturbatory act is the equivalent of losing forty drops of blood; that, if a girl does not bleed the first time she is penetrated vaginally in a sexual encounter, she is not a virgin; that sex during menstruation can make a man ill—all of these and so many other, similar notions are simply nonsense, but the folklore goes on. Some religions add to the problems induced by folkloric "wisdom" by listing masturbation, lack of virginity in a bride, and sex during menstruation as evils or sins or offenses against the divine will. How does one find a way through the maze? How does one approach the theme of human sexuality with an awareness of the direct and indirect influence of the Bible?

In this book an attempt is made to look at many of the ideas about human sexuality found in the Bible. Some Bible passages will be analyzed, utilizing methods and insights from literary, historical, and cultural studies. In some instances the biblical passages will be set in the larger framework of the ancient Near East and references will be made to the belief systems of surrounding nations. At other times, the focus will be on Hebrew, Jewish, and Christian communities only. The primary emphasis will be on the period extending from about 1100 Before the Common Era (B.C.E.) to about 150 of the Common Era (C.E.), the years in which the biblical materials were recorded. Then a leap will be made to the modern era. What does this literature, which is between 2,000 and 3,000 years old, have to offer to our present understanding of human sexuality? The question will require reference to psychological and sociological research, and at times there will be emphasis on therapeutic issues.

The limited use of Hebrew and Greek should not confuse the reader but will, it is hoped, elucidate particular meanings of words. The translations are, for the most part, my own. Where one of the newer translations of the Bible, or when some scholar has developed a felicitous phrase, I have not hesitated to use it.

Some statements may offend some Jews and Christians. One can only have respect for the belief systems of the various Jewish groups and the many different Christian denominations. The intent is not to offend, but to recognize that, despite the convictions of these groups and their particular understanding of what their scriptures mean and how they should be interpreted, there is room for differing opinions and interpretations and emphases, and perhaps also room for some judgmental statements about the scriptural interpretations made by these groups. At no point in this book is there a denial of the great contributions Jewish and Christian organizations in their various interpretations of their respective scriptures have made and continue to make to our culture and to the individual lives of the believers. At the same time, there can be no ignoring the fact that these same interpretations do not always work for human welfare, nor do they always enhance the individual.

Little of the material presented here will be new to clergy trained in accredited universities and seminaries by highly qualified instructors. If there is any complaint to be laid on their pastoral doorsteps, it is that they have failed to be educators and have not shared with their congregations the best results of the critical analysis of the Bible. As a result, they have produced and are continuing to produce parishioners who are either biblically naïve or biblical illiterates, able to be swayed and convinced by any Bible-thumping preacher who can raise the money to voice a particular interpretation through the electronic media. They are not equipped to challenge ideas or to research materials. They are told they must believe because the preachment is from "the word of God."

What kinds of attitudes toward sex are to be found in the Bible? Some biblical passages suggest that sex is a rather unsavory subject. Some sections set forth taboos and warn us against doing what might seem to come naturally lest we offend the deity. On the other hand, there are some erotic portions that express warm approval of sex, and here sex is presented as normal, natural, and desirable and no divine approval or disapproval is voiced—sex is just there to be enjoyed. Of course neither the synagogue nor the church have been willing to leave the interpretation of these passages to the average reader—someone might get the wrong idea! So it came to pass that religious leaders decided that the Song of Songs (and this is where the erotic material appears) could not represent human love—the passionate desire of a man for a woman and a woman for a man, a desire of the flesh. These leaders decided that what might appear to be the reflection of human love was in reality an expression of divine love—the love of the Hebrew deity Yahweh for his people Israel, or, if one prefers the Christian interpretation, the love of Christ for his church. The absurdity of this interpretation is immediately apparent to even the most casual reader. One must force the interpretation and, when fleshly passions surface, keep repeating, "This is the love of Yahweh for Israel!" or "This is the love of Christ for the church!" But more of this later.

The scholarly urge to overload the chapters with footnotes has been resisted more or less successfully and references have been reduced to but a few for certain sections. A small but important bibliography of easily accessible books appears at the end, and here some of the source materials can be found. Those interested in biblical interpretations are urged to go to their local public libraries and look into the *Interpreter's Dictionary of the Bible;* almost all of the articles in it are first rate. There are also some good commentaries on the market, and these too can be found in most good community libraries. None is difficult to read. The Anchor Bible commentaries are an excellent series of presentations by competent scholars in clear, readable English.

Most of all there is a need for clear thinking. Jews and Christians need to ask themselves "Does what the Bible has to say on this particular issue really have any importance or make any sense for someone living in the closing years of the twentieth century?" and "What makes me believe that those Jews and Christians who lived between 2,000 and 3,000 years ago knew more about human sexuality than our modern sex-researchers, therapists, and medical practitioners who give their whole lives to the study of the human body and its responses (albeit these persons can make errors too!)?" In other words, there is a need for common sense as well as a good deal of rational, logical analysis.

This book begins with the concept of the family and sex in the family. It moves on to what biblical writers (and some present-day people) consider to be deviations from the accepted norm. At times, certain ideas are repeated and certain biblical passages are used two or more times, often for emphasis or clarification, more often because a different theme is being explored and the passage casts light on the subject.

At this point it seems wise to issue a disclaimer. This is not a book of theology, but from time to time theological insights will be recognized. It is not a book of therapy, but implications of ideas for therapeutic work are acknowledged and therapeutic insights are introduced. It is a book that seeks to explore some of the ways in which biblical attitudes toward human sexuality impinge on our culture and have an impact on our individual lives.

1

The Family

The Family in Biblical Times

Studies of the ancient Hebrew family have found reminiscences of fratriarchies (where the eldest brother is the head of the family) and matriarchies (where a child's lineage is traced through the mother), but there can be little question that the dominant Hebrew family structure was patriarchal. Lineage was traced through the father. The nearest relative in the familial line was the paternal uncle (Lev. 25:49). The husband was the master (*ba'al*) of his wife because he activated her and caused her to bear children, and he had absolute authority over his children, including, at some period of early history, the power of life and death.

The family was not a nuclear one, but extended to include those united by a common bloodline as well as family slaves and servants, resident aliens, and family widows and orphans. Ideally all were under familial protection and, if harm came to one, it was harm to the total group. If the harm required repayment by an act of vengeance it was the responsibility of the *go'el*, the redeemer or rescuer or next of kin, to repay the debt. Vengeance could be in the form of a vendetta, such as that threatened by the Lamech group (Gen. 4:23–24) and that carried out by Dinah's brothers after she was raped (Gen. 34), or it could be one-to-one revenge, as when Absalom killed his half-brother Ammon for the rape of Tamar (2 Sam. 13).

Marriages were arranged by members of the family or their official representatives. The family of the marriageable man sought a suitable young woman. Agreements were reached between the parents or their official delegates. A marriage price (*mohar*) was paid by the man to the woman's family, partially as a recompense for the loss of a daughter and partially to compensate for the loss of power to her family because any children she might bear would strengthen her husband's family. The amount of *mohar* varied with the status of the woman and with the man's ability to pay. For example, when David wanted to marry King Saul's daughter Michal, David was a staff member in the palace and could not afford the kind of *mohar* such an alliance would ordinarily command. Saul permitted him to pay the price in Philistine foreskins (1 Sam. 18:17–29).

Young couples did meet one another and fall in love and make arrangements for marriage. Michal, Saul's daughter, loved David. Jacob loved Rachel (Gen. 29:18). But in most marriages the groom did not see the bride until after the marriage was consummated. Rebecca, who was chosen for Isaac by a servant of Abraham, remained veiled until they were married (Gen. 24:65–67). The man took the veiled woman to their home in the evening, and in the darkness copulated with her. It was not until morning that he could actually see her. In this way, Jacob's uncle, Laban, was able to substitute Leah, his older daughter, for Rachel, whom Jacob preferred (Gen. 29:23 ff.).

Weddings were occasions for the exchange of gifts. When the marriage arrangements were complete, the bride's family received *mohar* and gifts (Gen. 24:53). The father of the bride might give a special wedding gift to the new son-in-law. Solomon received the city of Gezer from Pharaoh when he married an Egyptian princess (1 Kings 9:16). The daughter, too, might receive gifts from her parents (Gen. 24:53; 29:24, 29). She would bring her dowry into the marriage, and it would be uniquely hers to keep and dispose of as she wished.

In most marriages the couple joined the husband's living group. There are a few exceptions. One in particular was the marriage of Samson to a Philistine woman who continued to live with her parents. Samson was expected to visit her from time to time (Judg. 14:1–15). This form of marriage is sometimes labeled a *sadiqa* (lover) marriage.

Both men and women married at a young age. It has been estimated that some of the members of the royal families (whose lengths of reign and other details are given in the books of Kings) married as young as fourteen (Amon and Josiah) or sixteen (Jehoiachin). As we shall see, some men were considerably older. It is assumed that the girls married quite young—just beyond puberty. Incestuous marriages were outlawed (as we shall see), but some marriages were entered into by first cousins. Mixed marriages did take place, but were not encouraged. The purpose of marriage was to raise a family, preferably consisting mostly of males. Should a man die without offspring, his brother was expected to copulate with his widow and produce a child in the dead man's name (see Chapter 3). Sex outside of marriage was forbidden and there were punishments for fornication and adultery.

As we shall see there was a clear-cut distinction between the significance of men and women. Males were more important, more valuable, and freer than women. A woman fulfilled herself in bearing children for her husband and in supporting him in whatever he was engaged in. She was to make the man happy, to fulfill his sexual needs, and to follow his lead. Women had little social standing and decisions were made by the men. There can be little doubt that many women exercised more authority than appeared on the surface because of their influence over the man in the home. Women used anger, sulking, and a bitter tongue to make their wishes known, but the ideal was always the submissive woman.

One might wonder what the effect of planned marriages might have been on the intimate relationships between husband and wife. In parts of the Arab world, planned marriages are still common. A brother or the father and brother together seek out a suitable woman for the eligible bachelor. They inquire into her education, her attitudes, her virtue. Once the agreement has been reached with her family and the *mahr* (the equivalent of *mohar*) has been paid, the marriage takes place with much celebration, often in the evening with the bride heavily veiled. The married couple go to their new home to discover one another. As one Jordanian gentleman put it as he enthusiastically embraced his brother: "This is my brother and I love him because he chose my beautiful wife for me. In your country you fall in love and marry; in my country we marry and fall in love. Who can say which is best?"

The arranged marriage is fading in the Near East as Western ideas in books, movies, and television influence the thinking of young people. Divorce is often American-style with legal settlements that give more protection to the woman than did the older pattern, which permitted the husband to give his wife a bill of divorce (Deut. 24:1, 3; Jer. 3:8; and elsewhere).

In the early Christian church, the concept of the family was not distinctly different from that of the Jewish community. The male was still the dominant authority figure. Wives were still expected to be submissive. As we shall see, some dimensions of sexual relationships are touched upon in Christian Scriptures, but it was generally in terms of the belief that the end of time was near and Jesus was soon to return and establish the Christian Kingdom of God. Hence everything had a "time" factor implied, including whether or not one should get married, the importance of sexual relationships, and so on. Some of these ideas will surface in subsequent discussion.

The many dimensions of biblical marriage and sexual relations will occupy the remainder of this book. Meanwhile, it is important to recognize how far removed we are from the ancient biblical world, and at the same time be aware of the impact of that world upon our present culture.

The Modern Family

We are a long distance from the biblical ideas about family. The ideal of father, mother, and children living happily together in a vine-covered cottage has not been lost; the vision is still there, but the reality is something different.[1] Although there are many couples who marry, buy a home, raise children, and remain faithfully married for the rest of their lives, the number of such families is diminishing. This is not because Westerners are forsaking the Bible and biblical mores, nor, as the so-called Moral Majority and ultra-right Christians would have us believe, because of the insidious teaching of humanism, but because of economic and social changes that are influencing family life.

At the beginning of the twentieth century most Western families consisted of a working father, a stay-at-home mother, and two or more children. Through good times and bad times, through family strife and family peace, the family often stayed together because divorce was not socially acceptable. This family structure was an important factor in the American industrial economy because it contributed reliable, disciplined male workers for the factories.

We are at a different place now. Nearly two-thirds of our labor force is involved in the production of information and services, and the economy is geared to this kind of business rather than to the industrial manufacturing economy of the past. Mothers no longer stay at home. In 1940, of all mothers with children under eighteen only 10 percent were working at jobs outside the home; by 1960 the number was 30 percent; today it is 55 percent. Whereas at the turn of the century children were almost always raised by both of their parents, today more and more are being brought up by only one. Indeed, the fastest-growing form of "family" in the United States today is the one-parent, female-headed family, of which there are now more than eight million. Lifelong monogamy has for some been replaced by what sociologists are calling "serial monogamy." One out of three marriages now ends in divorce (three times as many as in 1960), and over one-fifth of all marriages now involve one previously divorced person. As a result of the continuing patterns of separation and divorce and the growth in female-headed families, almost 45 percent of children born today can expect to live with only one parent by the time they are eighteen years of age. According to the 1981 census 12.6 million American children are living with one parent or with one natural parent and one step-parent. The majority, 48 million, live with both natural parents, and 2.2 million with neither parent. Many have no brothers or sisters, because the birthrate has dropped to 1.8 children from each woman's "fertility span"—a decline of 40 percent in just twenty years. Seventeen percent of married couples have no children.

Traditionally, in accordance with Jewish and Christian belief-systems, sex was supposed to take place only within marriage. Today there is evidence that in 1983 the number of couples who are living together outside of wedlock has tripled since 1970, and the number of adults who say that they approve of premarital intercourse rose from 20 percent in 1960 to more than 50 percent in 1980. Even among the many individuals between the ages of twenty-five and thirty-four who list themselves as "living alone" many are not chaste, sleep-alone persons. As a result there is a soaring rate of out-of-wedlock births. In 1979, nearly one in three white teen-agers and more than four out of five black teen-agers who gave birth were unmarried, according to an analysis of Census Bureau figures. In the past, more teen-agers gave up their babies for adoption; now, according to a 1978 study for the Planned Parenthood Federation of America, Inc., 96 percent of unwed teen-agers keep their babies. It has been estimated that some 597,800 out-of-wedlock babies were born in America in 1979, constituting 17 percent of all births, marking a significant increase from 1970, when out-of-wedlock births were 10.7 percent.

Sexual preferences that were once concealed, such as homosexuality, are now openly admitted. Attempts to legislate against oral sex have been laughed out of legislative bodies. Recreational sex has become more popular. It is as though the replacement by the Reagans of the portrait of Thomas Jefferson in the White House by that of Calvin Coolidge is a tacit although perhaps unwitting recognition of the so-called "Coolidge Effect" as a functioning reality in present society. The Coolidge Effect is based on a report of a field trip to a poultry station taken by President and Mrs. Coolidge sometime between 1923 and 1927. The group was so large that it was divided into two parts, and the President and Mrs. Coolidge inspected the station separately, with Mrs. Coolidge's group leading. When her group reached a particular yard where the rooster was working vigorously at his task of impregnating a large flock of hens, Mrs. Coolidge asked the technician in charge, "Does he perform like that all day?" When she was assured that this was so, the First Lady said, "Indeed! Please point him out to the President." When the President arrived at the same yard, the technician conveyed the message. Mr. Coolidge asked, "And does he regularly change females?" On being assured that this was so, the President responded, "Indeed! Please tell that to Mrs. Coolidge."

The point of the Coolidge Effect is that polygamous animals may be roused sexually by changing partners. Experiments among animal breeders and zoo keepers have tended to verify this hypothesis. The idea that monogamy leads to sexual boredom may not lie behind the nonmarital, extramarital, nonprocreative sex boom, but changes in the social structure, the development of more effective birth-control methods, and the freeing of women from traditional roles of house-keeper and nursemaid, have made the opportunities for exploring the validity of the Coolidge Effect available to millions of people. The changes reflect the new social and economic patterns. The composition of the labor force changed after World War II. Not only had women responded to a national crisis by taking jobs during wartime, but they experienced something of their own potentials in work that had not been open to them before. Employers responded to the availability of nonunionized female labor for jobs in offices, stores, restaurants, schools, and health facilities. Older women with grown children took jobs. Then, with the coming of inflation, women with growing children in the family recognized the need for extra funds for higher education, and they too became involved. Young married couples, needing money for down-payments on homes, delayed having children as both worked. After the first child came, the wife returned to work to help maintain the family standard of living.

The religious ultra-right continues to call for a return to the life-style of a former age. Like the prophets in ancient Israel who kept demanding that the nation return to the patterns of the desert sojourn, these Christian conservatives, some of whom call themselves the "Moral Majority," are just as out of touch with social and economic realities as were the prophets of old—except when it comes to collecting money from those whom they try to frighten with their portents of doom. These conservatives, who are in reality a minority, are troubled by changes in

American family life and social mores. They do not see that these changes are not the deliberate creations of depraved humanists but represent human responses to systemic changes, including shifts in the sexual composition of the labor force. If they had their way, women would be put back in the kitchen and our developing capitalism would be shifted into reverse. There are new horizons developing in economic and sexual behavior. To insist that we accept biblical patterns, as these religious conservatives would have us do, is to be out of touch with the growth patterns within our culture and throughout the world. The Bible contains many inspiring moral statements, and some of these statements are meaningful to our present age. But each claim made by the fundamentalists needs to be examined in the light of biblical exegesis and research and with an awareness of the implications for individual life and growth. The family structure is in the process of change; sexual patterns are changing, too.

Resistance to change also comes from other conservative religious groups, and sometimes they are compelled to yield to better ideas. For example, until 1981 Greece was the only European country where adultery was still a penal offense. Unfaithful husbands and wives used to be bundled up in blankets and taken naked to the police station, where adultery charges could result in imprisonment for up to one year. The strongest opposition to changing these laws came from the Greek Orthodox church. Because of the Greek church's attitude toward adultery, those who divorced after such a charge are barred from remarriage; as a result, couples live together unwed and produce children who are labeled "illegitimate." More women than men have been sentenced for adultery in Greece, because women seldom take such charges against their husbands to court for fear of losing the prized social status of being a married woman. Divorced women have little chance of remarriage in Greece.

Sometimes religious groups only reaffirm their conservative stance. In December 1981, Pope John Paul II, in an "apostolic exhortation," or letter to the clergy, reaffirmed the Roman Catholic church bans on divorce, abortion, polygamy, trial marriage, and contraception. The fact that 76.5 percent of Roman Catholic couples in the United States are reported to be using contraceptives did not deter the pope, who is reported to have said "the truth is not always the same as majority opinion." The pope urged the clergy to correct with charity those living together out of wedlock and to help them "regularize" the situation. He urged pastors to treat those Catholics married outside of the church with the same charitable spirit and to urge them to "regularize" their situation so that they might partake of the sacraments from which they are banned. Those divorced Catholics who remarry are also banned from the sacraments unless they live "in complete continence, that is, by abstinence from acts proper only to married couples."[2]

It is also clear that new insights into marriage relationships, when they are heeded by the public and encouraged by the clergy, can help couples develop long-term, lasting marriages. Such marriages require "working at." Problems must be faced day by day and worked through rationally, with deep appreciation and respect for the rights and feelings of each person. The models provided by couples who have achieved ''golden age'' marriages that have lasted for up to fifty years and more can give some guidance. They indicate that commitment to each other and to working through their problems, as well as the lack of desire or an unwillingness to be with anyone else, made it possible for couples to stay together despite the ups and downs of life. Other studies have concentrated on the dramatic changes that take place in families when children leave home, or when the man retires and the woman continues to work, or when the man retires and is then free to putter about the house that was the woman's domain up to that time. These midlife crises can be met and overcome if the couple is willing to work through the problems, often with the help of trained marriage and family counselors. Many religious organizations structure weekend retreats where couples can come together and, through a guided program, rediscover one another. For many the results are beneficial and contribute to the growth and stability of the relationship.

NOTES

1. Material in this section is drawn primarily from an article by Marvin Harris, Graduate Research Professor of Anthropology at the University of Florida and author of *America Now: The Anthropology of a Changing Culture* (New York, 1981). The article was printed in the *Los Angeles Times*, December 23, 1981.

2. Associated Press report from the Vatican in the *Los Angeles Times*, December 16, 1981.

2

Sex Education

Evangelical Christians and members of the religious far-right in all denominations continually criticize the sex-education courses offered in public schools. They are appalled at the texts and films that show the naked body and explain the sexual functions of the genitals. Pictures showing live births are condemned with the same words and in the same tone as those used in protests against pornography. The negative results of such education are estimated by these protesters in terms of the increased number of teen-age abortions and practice of birth-control and the rise in premarital sex. Opponents of sex education argue that the Bible and ''the Christian concept of the family'' are the paramount issues and that sex should be learned in the home from parents.

Surveys have shown how little children learn about sex from their parents. Either the parents are too embarrassed to talk explicitly about the sex organs and reproduction or they are poorly informed. One twenty-one-year-old Mormon woman, about to be married, admitted that although she had been raised in the church in Utah and had attended church-related educational institutions (she had a bachelor's degree in science), she knew very little about her own body, less about the body of her fiancé, and possessed only the vaguest notions about sexual relations. Her homelife had been warm, but physical expressions of affection were eschewed. She had never seen her father hug or kiss her mother. She desired warmth and affection, but found herself rather stiff and awkward and a bit uncomfortable when her fiancé held her ''too close'' or ''too long.'' She fantasized a family life like that of her parents. ''They obviously knew what to do and how to make love, they had nine children,'' she said. She was insecure about entering into the sexual life of marriage. ''But,'' she said, ''he's the man and he will know what to do!''

There is no doubt that many couples establish a married life and raise a family with a limited knowledge of their own bodies and with only a casual understanding of sexual intimacies. They learn by doing, and often from their learning they hit upon a satisfactory way of expressing their love sexually. On the other hand, the constant stream of disaffected couples that seek counseling for marriages that are marred by inadequate sexual responses, by lack of knowledge of each other's needs, wishes, and desires, and by misinformation can only represent the tip of an iceberg of sexual discontent and of marital disharmony related to sex. Perhaps sex education would not provide the solution to all marital or sexual problems, but certainly some of the problems stemming from misinformation and lack of information might be eliminated.

The attempt to correlate the rise in abortions or the increase in promiscuous sex with courses in sex education is simply unconvincing. Nor can the humanist movement be singled out as a contributing factor. Promiscuous sex has always been part of the human scene and the condemnation of violation of established mores can be found in biblical literature and in the literature of cultures both ancient and modern. That there has been an increase of premarital sexual activity has also been well documented, and this increase suggests that modern youths and adults are challenging traditional Jewish and Christian teachings about sex. Books, films, better education, wider reading, faster and better exchange of information, the changing pattern of the family with the increase of the freedom of children from parental supervision, extended travel, the acquisition of knowledge about the attitudes of different cultures to sexual behavior have had a profound effect on modern young people. They are aware of human sexuality. They are curious about their bodies and body response. They are not compelled to avoid questions; modern education encourages inquiry. They want to know about their bodies and about sex, and if they do not get good information and guidance from the schools they may get inadequate data the way some of their parents got it—from poorly informed peers, in back-alley sessions, or smirking or giggling schoolboy and schoolgirl exchanges. Children are better informed now than ever before; but there are still far too many who are ill informed.

What youths do with this knowledge is a completely different matter. There can be no question that in families where high moral standards and strong ethical values are taught and practiced the children will tend to live by these learned standards. But, because standards are constantly in flux, they may not accept everything that their parents have taught. They may fall in love with someone from a different country, representing a different race or religious background. There may be discrepancies in age that are not in accord with parental beliefs about what the age-range of husband and wife should be. One partner may have been married before and there may be a ready-made family. But what is most important in any marriage is the quality of the relationship, including tenderness and tolerance, showing and expressing love and concern, acquiring a healthy balance between protectiveness and freedom, maintaining respect for the rights of each member of the family—all of these factors, and more.

Studies have shown that most often the mother is the primary source of sex education but that regardless of whether this education was received from the father or the mother the fact that the initial learning was in a familial setting tends to result in the initiation into sex taking place at a later age and with fewer premarital partners. Where the fourteen- to sixteen-year-old daughter's socio-emotional needs were met by maternal support and communication, there was less likelihood of the daughter seeking intimate relationships as a means to fulfill or meet socio-emotional needs. Nonvirgins were found to have poorer communication with their mothers than virgins have. The mother's past and current marital and nonmarital sexual activities were also found to provide role models for their teen-aged daughters. There can be no doubt that family solidity and the belief systems and value orientation of the family can have nourishing effects on the lives of the children.

But the statistics also reveal how poor the communication is in many families and how inadequate sex education is, despite the excellence of school programs. More is needed. Thirty percent of our children are having their first sex experience when they are between the ages of thirteen and fifteen. In the sixteen- to eighteen-year-old group it is 60 percent. Only 14 percent of teen-agers seek birth-control advice before their first sexual experience. Seventy-three percent of sexually active teen-aged girls have never attempted any method of birth control. Some will acknowledge that they have heard of a diaphragm; few have ever seen one. They know about condoms, but if the boy hasn't got one they go ahead anyway.

The results of this massive lack of sex information are impressive. Every day three thousand teen-aged girls become pregnant. Each year unmarried teen-aged girls have babies. The sharpest increase in births is among girls under fourteen. How well a thirteen-year-old boy who fathers a child and a thirteen-year-old girl who bears the child are equipped to take care of an infant when they are little more than children themselves can only be imagined. The baby may be kept by the young mother and her family or be put up for adoption. Unless the two thirteen-year-old parents are given proper sex education, it is quite possible they will engage in sexual intercourse again with similar results—they are simply too young to grasp the ramifications of what they are about without help. There are now more than five million babies living with teen-aged mothers who have not completed high school. These young mothers move out from their family homes and attempt to cope with life. Because they have no education, they can't get jobs and so must rely upon public welfare. In their frustration they may abuse their children. Some move in with men from whom they hope to get love and protection, and many find only abuse for themselves and their infants. Many of the girls are under sixteen when they give birth. At eighteen they have a toddler underfoot and they have still not graduated from high school. The result is a whole class of infants born to and living with mothers who are poorly educated. Because they know no other life, these infants will tend to grow and follow the models they find in their mothers.

The need for sex education is clear. To attempt to block it is a call to deny what is happening in our country. To blame humanism is naive. To insist that one must turn to the Bible for sexual education is to attempt to go back in time two thousand to three thousand years and to argue that the slim record of religious literature that is accepted from that ancient period is enough to provide modern children with adequate information about love and procreation. The notion is a stupid one; it reflects a lack of knowledge about what the Bible teaches and a denial of what is happening in modern society.

To insist that sex education be provided only by parents is to fail to recognize the inadequacy of many parents to provide proper information and to ignore the feelings of embarrassment some adults feel when they attempt to talk about sex. Most parents are ill equipped to transfer the best information on this important subject.

Should there be courses in sex education in the churches? Some church groups do provide sex education as part of their youth training programs. Most of the time the information is not specific and is comparable to what a student might get in a general biology lecture. Nor are many church-school instructors well enough trained to deal with the subject unless they have had courses in sex education, preferably at the college level, and have read widely on the subject. As we shall see, it is one thing to talk about "the evils of homosexuality," it is another to deal compassionately with the burdens society places on the gay population and to understand that the attraction to members of the same sex may be a natural (in church terms, God-given) characteristic of some individuals.

Finally, there must be some questions raised about the Bible as an adequate tool for sex education. Some of the biblical superstitions about certain aspects of the body (menstruation, for example) are really not relevant to modern life and are only recognized by the most extreme orthodox followers. We have come a long way scientifically since the biblical texts were written, and youth needs to be prepared for life in this time period. Some of the mores and values set forth in the Bible are still significant—but not because they are promulgated by ancient Israel or ancient Christians—the values are human values and belong to humans in all times and places. The particular sexual values of the Bible may or may not apply to some groups in modern society—most Jews and Christians are selective in what they choose to follow. But something more than the Bible is needed, and well-planned, well-taught courses in sexual education fill part of that need.

Sex Education in Ancient Israel

There was sex education in ancient Israel, just as there is sex education in every culture. How good, how effective, how humane, how sensitive and warm the emphasis is in each setting can only be determined by the values placed upon the individual—the status, value, importance, significance, and worth of each person, including the young and the old, the male and the female, the native-born and the alien. The Bible portrays cultural patterns in which the male is more important than the female, the native-born more important than the alien, the followers of Yahweh or Jesus more important than those who were outside of these belief systems, the parent more important than the child and male children more important than female.

What was sex education like in the ancient world? How did boys and girls learn about procreation? Where did they learn to make love? Where did they learn the language of love? The techniques of love-making? The ways of tenderness and caring?

As far as we can tell there were no formal courses in sex education provided by the royal court, the temple, the synagogue, or the early church in biblical times. Children learned about sex by observation. No doubt youngsters got together and shared their information. Just as modern youths learn about sex from their environment today—from television, movies, radio, magazines and books, conversations with other youths, and in some cases from answers given by adults to their questions—so the youth of ancient Palestine would learn about sex from their environment.

Archaeological research has shown that the communities in the ancient world tended to be small, self-contained units consisting of houses clustered together within a walled village, town, or city. Streets were narrow and were sometimes cobbled. There were no toilet facilities and no baths or running water in the homes. There was little privacy. The smallest units consisted of a single room with a walled courtyard in front. Most homes were small two- or three-room structures facing a walled courtyard. Some were "L"-shaped, with the open part of the "L" forming the court. Some may have had two-stories. Both the single-story and two-story houses had provision for using the rooftop for sleeping and for other activities during the hot weather. Wealthier families might have had two-story houses built around an open atrium, but most could not afford such luxury. Food would be cooked in the courtyard and some food may have been kept there in large storage jars. During inclement weather, one room would be used for cooking and storing food. Another room, sometimes constructed separately, but often included within the home proper, would house animals at night and during stormy weather. One room would be set aside as sleeping quarters for the family, although in larger homes and in wealthier families the children might be separated from the adults.

The houses were built of stone with flat, wooden roofs sealed with clay or plaster. Floors were plastered and may have been covered in part by rugs or woven mats. Furnishings were simple.

While there were certainly markets in each community, meat did not come in plastic wrappings and was not preserved in a deep-freeze. Animals were bred and killed for food. Children would witness what few modern children see, the mating of animals. This may be a crude form of "sex education," but from earliest childhood the mounting of the female by the male would be witnessed by almost every child; and the importance of this mating act for the increase of flocks and herds would be known to every child. They would understand that at certain times animals were in "heat" and the female was eager to receive the male. The prophet Jeremiah knew he would be understood by every listener when he described apostate Israel in its participation in the Canaanite fertility cults as "a wild ass . . . in her heat sniffing the wind" (Jer. 2:24).

Urination by males was never a secret or private affair. Several biblical passages refer to the male as the one who "pisses" against the wall—a custom that is still practiced in some Near-East communities and, even if it is not always observed, the aromatic reality can be attested to on a hot day! (Compare 1 Sam. 25:22, 34; 1 Kings 14:10; 16:11; 21:21; 2 Kings 9:8.) Modern translations prefer to use the term "urinate" or perhaps avoid any reference to the act by translating "he who pisseth against the wall" of the King James version as "every mother's son" (New English Bible). The numerous references to "shit" or "dung" make it clear that there was a crude bluntness in language among the common people just as there is today.

There could be no true bodily privacy in the ancient household. Bathing of children by parents would be a family affair. Children would become aware of differences in genitals at an early age. Although parents might bathe privately (how often cannot be known), young women would learn from their mothers of the need to bathe after menstruation according to Jewish religious law and would therefore learn something of the bodily functions and of the restrictions concerning intercourse during the menstrual period (Lev. 15:19 ff.; 20:18).

Sleeping arrangements put bodies in close proximity, making it a simple matter for boys and girls to become aware of their genital differences. It is doubtful that children slept more soundly in the ancient past than they do today, and it is also doubtful that sexual intercourse was any quieter than it is today. In the closeness of the sleeping quarters, body movement, harsh breathing, panting, and even cries of pleasure could not be hidden, even through thick stone walls. Nocturnal intercourse could not have been as private as it is in many homes today. Then, too, it is quite possible that during the afternoon the parents would send the children to play away from home, the mother would don her finest garb and dance for her husband before they engaged in coitus. The pattern is not unknown among Arab villagers in Palestine today.

When a child was born, there was no sterile hospital to cater to the physical and emotional needs of the mother. Midwives attended the mother to assist in the birth, to comfort and advise (Gen. 35:17; 38:28; Exod. 1), and children were born at home. The labor cries of the mother could be heard by all members of the family and possibly by those in neighboring houses. Micah 4:10 capitalizes on the common knowledge of how a woman in labor responds as she gives birth and the Psalmist could also make reference to the same experience (Ps. 48:6; see also Jer. 4:31; 6:24; 22:23; etc.). Procreation, birth, and family intimacies could not be hidden from the growing child.

Fertility-Cult Centers

Within each village there were shrines associated with fertility. At this moment it is impossible to reconstruct exactly what rites and observances were performed there, but from the condemnation by the prophets and from the numerous folk tales in the Bible it is obvious that sexual interaction was part of the cult. So powerful and so prominent were these cultic ceremonies that Jeremiah could speak of total family involvement. He stated that "the children gather the wood, the fathers start the fire and the women prepare the dough to bake cakes for the queen of heaven, and they pour out drink offerings to other gods" (Jer. 7:18). The queen of heaven was Ishtar, her symbol was the evening star, and the cakes made in her honor were star-shaped (Jer. 44:19). The worship rites associated with this goddess and with the Canaanite deities included fertility symbols such as a stone and a tree that could be addressed as parents (Jer. 2:27). The rites involved intercourse. Male and female cult prostitutes served their gods at the shrines. When worshipers engaged in intercourse with these cult prostitutes, they participated in an act of holy communion with the god or goddess, stimulating the deity to act beneficently and grant prosperity in the form of agricultural success. Jeremiah claimed that the Hebrew men performed sexually with these prostitutes on every hilltop and under any green tree (Jer. 2:20). Amos condemned the man and his son who copulated with the same cult prostitute and lay down on clothing that had been contributed to the shrine (Amos 2:7–8). The fertility shrines must have provided the growing children in Hebrew villages with additional knowledge of sexual behavior.

In cultic festivals, the clergy reenact the myths of the faith, either symbolically or in actuality. In our present culture, Jews use symbols at Pesach to reenact the Passover story. Children are involved in the recitation of certain lines, food calls to mind the wilderness sojourn, and adults celebrate and emphasize freedom. Christians reenact the crucifixion and the resurrection. On Good Friday, the church furnishings are draped in somber colors and the emphasis is upon sacrificial death. In Jerusalem pilgrims carry a heavy cross down the Via Dolorosa. On Easter Sunday, all is transformed. The church is arrayed in bright colors with symbols of new life. Easter fare marks a celebration; sermons emphasize resurrection. Children take part in Easter-egg hunts. There may be a dramatization of the empty tomb or an early morning walk to some hillock topped with a cross to reenact the role of the women who went to the empty tomb. So, too, in the ancient cults the rites reenacted the stories about the deities.

Canaanite and Mesopotamian myths recorded the sexual exploits of the deities. To what extent these were physically enacted before the local people or how explicit the enactment was cannot be determined. Certainly the myths could be told and symbolically dramatized.

The terms of endearment and language of love used by the gods who were lovers and sexual partners has been recovered from ancient Sumer and Ugarit. It is not unlike the language of the Song of Songs in the Bible; it is sensuous, warm, and tender. It evokes images of caressing and feelings of intimacy. It is believed that these were the words used in the fertility rites to express the way in which divine lovers approached and responded to one another. Indeed, the Song of Songs, which contains no mention of God, was a controversial book. It got into the Jewish canon because (according to Rabbi Akiba and his followers) it did not represent human love but Yahweh's love for Israel. Later the Christian church argued that it represented Christ's love for his church. One need only read the book with either of these allegorical approaches in mind to see immediately how absurd the interpretation is. Some scholars have found parallels between modern Syrian wedding songs and the Song of Songs. It seems probable that the poems in the Song of Songs came out of the ancient fertility cult of Canaan and that Syrian wedding songs are reminiscent of these same ancient fertility rites.

If the language of the fertility cult poems of ancient Sumer and Canaan or of the Song of Songs are representative of what was said during the fertility rituals in ancient Palestine, the Hebrew youth would be educated in the tender language of love in a far more effective manner than modern youth may be through the violence so often associated with sex in the tabloids and on the screen.

Finally, the Bible itself documents the rich sexual religious heritage of ancient Palestine. The Hebrews entered from the desert into a well-established culture that recognized fertility religion as important to the environment. Christianity developed in the Greco-Roman world, which was rich in religions that had sexual overtones and where different kinds of sexual behavior were accepted. Communication may have lacked the speed of the modern world, but communities were small and less could be hidden even from the casual observer. Only by separation from the community, by isolation into tight little islands of religiosity, could those who lived in the ancient Near East be separated from the impact of normal, everyday human sexual behavior.

To be ignorant is one thing, to be innocent is another. Reliable, intelligent information is available in our modern environment, just as it was available in other contexts in ancient Israel. Whether one should accept the precepts of the Jews and Christians who lived 2,000 to 3,000 years ago as adequate for the last fifth of the twentieth century can be debated. Whether one accepts the Bible (no matter which collection of books or which translation) as the divinely inspired word of God, to be believed and followed in all details pertaining to faith and conduct, is a personal matter. The variety of Jewish and Christian organizations and the wide disparity in their handling of and interpreting their scriptures indicate that there is no final answer satisfactory to all. The Religious Right can insist that their children get sex education only from members of ultraconservative groups and not be compelled to take sex education in public classes. They do not have the right to prevent others from being educated.

The Schools of the Wise

Although so far as we know there was no formal sex-education course provided in ancient Israel, there was instruction for life provided by the wise men for their students. The teachings were not based on divine revelation, such as that claimed by the prophets or by the Torah; the wisdom was drawn from life, from observation. These older men had, so to speak, "been there." They had moved through life observing the behavior that brought disaster and the patterns that produced success. Their sayings have been gathered and belong in the literary category known as "wisdom" (hokmah). The collected sayings are something more than simple folk-wisdom such as that represented by the wise woman (hakmah) who was sent by Joab to repair the breach between David and Absalom. She, in her wisdom, used a parable to cause the monarch to rethink his position (2 Sam. 14:1–20). The teachings of the wise men were, presumably, used over and over again to provide instruction in wise and good living. They may have been taught formally in a school presided over by a sage.

Many scholars have accepted the idea that the royal court in Israel, beginning perhaps with David, but certainly with Solomon, established royal schools to train potential government employees. These schools, which would have been modeled on those in Egypt and Mesopotamia, educated young men of the upper-class families in the skills of writing, mathematics, and socially acceptable behavior. The teachers, the wise men, employed maxims, aphorisms, parables, and preachments to guide their young patrons about what behavior would lead to success and what promised failure. The young men would copy and recopy these maxims, acquiring both skill in writing and a set of guidelines for behavior.

Although the teachers did not ignore the theological aspects of Israel's religion, it was not central to their teaching. Their maxims were in accord with the accepted beliefs, but the teaching material was drawn from life experiences and from observation about how certain behavior affected the lives of individuals.

The teachings have been gathered together in the books of Proverbs, Ecclesiastes, the book of Job, the book of Ecclesiasticus, or "The Wisdom of Jesus, the son of Sirach" (which we will abbreviate to Sirach), and a first-century B.C.E. writing known as "The Wisdom of Solomon." Although some of the wisdom teachings appear to be products of a school, by the time of the beginning of Christianity learning centers had developed around single individuals. Such a school was run by Jesus, son of Sirach.

Almost universally the wise men extolled the virtues of honesty, humility before the powerful, diligence and hard work, loyalty and helpfulness. They warned against deceit, presumptuousness, slothfulness, unreliability, and indifference to social mores. They praised the benefits of marriage, although they warned their students that not all marriages were happy (Prov. 19:13; 21:19; 25:24; Sirach 25:16 ff.; 26:7). They set forth the qualities of the good wife the young men should look for. Good wives made their husbands happy (Prov. 31:10–31; Sirach 25:8; 26:1; 13–18), helped to train the children (Prov. 1:8–9), and rejoiced when their men succeeded and were sad when they failed (Prov. 10:1; 17:25; 23:25; 28:24). At a later time Christian wisdom expanded on the role of the woman. They were to recognize that they were secondary, in that they were made from men for men (1 Cor. 11:8). They were to remain silent in the churches and be aware of their secondary status. If they wished to get information, they asked their husbands at home (1 Cor. 14:33 ff). They were to dress modestly and sensibly without fancy hair arrangements or costume jewelry. They were to listen quietly and submissively and should recognize that their salvation came through child-bearing (1 Tim. 2).

The ancient wise men warned their students against evil, seductive women, because involvement with such persons could only lead to trouble. They were told that the way of wisdom would protect the youth from the wiles of

> the estranged [strange] woman,
> the non-conforming [foreign] woman
> with her smooth speech
>
> [Prov. 2:16]

The reference may be to the woman who has strayed from her husband or who has wandered away from acceptable social norms; but it may also be a warning against a woman who is a member of a foreign fertility cult—perhaps the cult of Ishtar, the Babylonian goddess of love, war, and fertility. Participation in foreign religious fertility rites could be interpreted as wasting the holy semen of an Israelite to produce offspring that would not strengthen the family. The young men are urged to

> drink water from your own cistern
> running water from your own well.
> Should your springs [semen?] be scattered outside?
> channels of water [semen?] in the streets?
> Let them be for yourself only,
> not for the strangers among you.
>
> [Prov. 5:15–17]

The same idea is echoed in a passage that is not found in all ancient manuscripts of Sirach. The sage is supposed to have warned:

> My son, guard the bloom of youth
> and do not waste your strength on strangers
> Look over the whole plain for a fertile plot
> then sow your seed [semen], trusting in your lineage,
> Your children will prosper in confidence of their parentage.
>
> [Sirach 26:19–21]

Both in Proverbs and in Sirach the tone is that of a father-to-son lecture providing man-to-man frank advisement. There is nothing preachy in the sayings that recommends sticking to one's own wife and not yielding to the temptation to become involved with other women. The advice is practical: not only can such involvement be costly in the loss of wealth and reputation, but it can lead to death.

A wise man in Proverbs set forth a tantalizing description of a wife for his young students. She was a lovely deer, "a graceful doe." The young man is urged to "let her breasts intoxicate you, be ravished by her love" (5:19). But temptations for young men seem to have been everywhere! The wise teacher related his experience as an observer of youthful folly:

> At the window of my house
> as I looked out through the lattice-work
> I saw among the young men
> noticed among the [immature] youths
> one senseless young man
> going along the street near her corner
> taking his way to her house,
> at twilight, in the evening, in the shadowy darkness of night.
> And look! a woman comes to meet him, dressed like a whore
> and heavily veiled
> she is wanton and rebellious and her feet do not stay at home
> Now she loiters in the streets at the corners
> She seizes him and kisses him and with brazen demeanor says to him,
> Today I must fulfill my vows and make a sacrificial meal
> So I have come to meet you, to seek out your face and I have found you
> I have spread on my bed coverlets
> of colored linen from Egypt,
> I have perfumed my bed
> with myrrh, aloes and cinnamon.
> Come let us saturate ourselves with love [in lust] till morning,
> let us completely fill ourselves with love;
> For my husband is not at home,
> he has gone on a long journey
> he has taken a bag of money with him,
> he will return home at full moon.
> With her seductive charms she entices him.
> with her persuasive words she lures him.
> suddenly he follows her,
> he goes like an ox to the slaughter . . .

[Prov. 7:6–22]

It is possible, as some commentators have suggested, that the woman is a devotee of Aphrodite or Ishtar, married to a wealthy businessman. Part of the fertility ritual involved a sacral meal and copulation. Others have argued that the fertility cult issue is insignificant, that the teacher is warning his students against involvement with a married woman who is acting like a whore, or who indeed may be a prostitute. There are ample warnings against such affairs in the words of the wise. The sage insisted that the wise words were designed to protect you from the evil woman

> from the smooth tongue of the alienated [foreigner?]
> Do not lust after her beauty
> Do not let her ensnare you with her eyelashes
> For a whore [can be had] for a round loaf of bread
> But a[nother] man's wife hunts with a costlier appetite.
> Can a man carry fire against his chest
> without burning his clothes?
> Or can a person walk on glowing coals
> without scorching his feet?
> So it is with the one who goes into [has intercourse with] his neighbor's wife;
> No one who touches her will go unpunished.
>
> [Prov. 6:24–29]

A wise man added, "He who commits adultery is senseless" (Prov. 6:32). Sirach also condemned "an old fool who commits adultery" (Sirach 25:2). He warned against

> A man who commits adultery in his own bed
> and says in his heart (thinks), "who sees me?"
> the walls of my house conceal me
> and the roof overshadows me
> so no one sees me
> so what is to hinder me from sinning?
>
> [Sirach 23:18]

He condemned the wanton wife:

> so too the wife who strays from her husband
> and conceives children by a stranger . . .
> . . . through her fornicating she has committed adultery
> and born children by another man.
> She will be led [for punishment] before the assembly
> and the punishment will be visited upon her children.
> Her children will not take root
> and her branches will bear no fruit . . .
>
> [Sirach 23:22]

The wise student avoided compromising situations with women. Sirach advised:

> Do not sit at the table (recline on your elbow) with
> another man's wife,
> And do not party with her with wine

[Sirach 9:9]

He continued:

> Wine and women fill the heart [mind] with lust
> and he who frequents with whores becomes reckless.
> Decay [sores?] and worms will possess him
> for his recklessness will destroy him.

[Sirach 19:2]

It is possible that Sirach is referring to some venereal disease, but it is equally possible that he means that the way of whores is the way of death. Agur ben Jakeh of Massa, whose words have been preserved in the book of Proverbs, described his observation of the adulteress:

> This is the act of an adulteress: she eats, wipes her mouth
> and declares: "I have done nothing wrong!"

[Prov. 30:20]

He may be speaking in general of the woman fulfilling her sexual appetite. His words suggest oral copulation.

Awareness of sexual relations was certainly part of the environmental education of youth in ancient Israel. The teachings about the evils of certain sexual acts or about certain associations may have kept some individuals away from what the faith labeled unacceptable. But violations did occur and, for some, breaking the accepted moral code must have produced guilt—guilt associated with feelings about sex, with sexual desires and fantasies as well as with any involvement in sex outside of marriage. The religious teachings, with their threats of punishment, must have engendered fear that the deity would punish and bring to pass the threatened doom and downfall predicted by the wise. The pattern has not changed. In a study made in 1964 Dr. James Peterson found that among the 420 married people studied, sex guilt was highest among those of conservative denominations and lowest among those with no religious affiliation.[1] Helping those burdened by guilt is a demanding therapeutic responsibility. Some kinds of sexual education engaged in by conservative religious groups may add burdens to those who engage in what those outside of the group accept as normal sexual behavior.

NOTE

1. James Peterson, *Education for Marriage* (New York, 1964).

3

The Levirate

A Hebrew law, for which parallels can be found in surrounding ancient nations, provides that if a man died without offspring it was the duty of his brother to copulate with the dead man's widow to produce offspring. The child born of such a union would bear the name of the dead man, would be considered to be his son, would keep the name of the dead man alive, and would inherit his property and provide status for the widow. The marriage has been called levirate or brother-in-law marriage (from Latin *levir* = husband's brother; Hebrew, *yabam*).

The continuation of the name was important because the Hebrews believed that, so long as a man's name was remembered, he continued to exist. Once the name was obliterated, it was as if he had never existed. The concept of the afterlife in early Israel did not include ideas of heaven and hell—these developed later. The shade of the individual continued a shadowy existence in the underworld (*Sheol*), but there was no personal immortality.

If a widow married outside of the family, the husband's property would be transferred to another man's family. Should she die without offspring, there was a chance that a slave might inherit. Levirate marriage protected the family property.

The Deuteronomic law reflects the ancient patterns:

When brothers live together and one of them dies without a son, his widow shall not marry outside of the family, but her husband's brother shall go to her and copulate with her [literally: brother-in-law her]. The first son she bears will be successor to the dead brother's name, so his name will not be blotted out of Israel. If the man does not wish to take his brother's wife, then the widow shall go to the elders at the [city] gate and declare, "My brother-in-law refuses to perpetuate his brother's name in Israel, he will not brother-in-law me." And the elders of the city shall summon him and counsel him, and if he persists and says, "I do not wish to take her," his sister-in-law shall approach him in the presence of the elders, remove his sandal from his foot and spit in his face, saying, "This is what is done to a man who will not build up his brother's family." And in Israel, his (family) name will be known as "The house of him who had his sandal removed." [Deut. 25:5–10]

The setting of the legislation is the extended family, where sons and daughters continue to live in the family household or dwell nearby, and where a younger brother might be housed with an older married brother. The court consisted of the elders who sat on low stone benches in the entryway to the town gate under the shadow of the protecting walls. It is clear that the brother-in-law was not required to take his brother's wife, but he was expected to make his decision known publicly and denial of that responsibility would label him and his offspring as something less than loyal.

The levirate regulation only surfaces a few times in biblical literature. The story of Ruth revolves around this ruling. A Bethlehemite family moved to Moab during a drought. While they were there, the two sons married Moabite women. Subsequently all of the men died. Naomi, the mother of the two young men decided to return to her home-town of Bethlehem, accompanied by one of her daughters-in-law, Ruth. They were in dire circumstances after their return, and Ruth went to the field to gather any stalks of grain the reapers might have missed. Boaz, the owner of the field, was attracted to her and ordered his reapers to leave substantial droppings of grain for Ruth.

When Naomi became aware of the man's interest in her daughter-in-law, she advised Ruth to "pretty herself up" and, when Boaz had fallen asleep on the threshing floor, to go and "uncover his feet." The word *feet* is a euphemism for "genitals" and there can be little doubt about the sexual connotations in the account. Naomi said that Boaz would tell Ruth "what to do." At midnight Boaz awakened to find a woman lying by his genitals. He spread his robe over her, which was a symbol of taking possession of her and of protective custody. He explained to her that there was a closer relative who had prior claim on her according to levirate law and that that man had to be consulted. The man refused to honor his obligation, the rite of removing his sandal was carried out, and Ruth and Boaz married and were the ancestors of King David.

A legend associated with the patriarch Judah also involves levirate marriage (Gen. 38). When Judah's son Er died without offspring, Onan, the brother-in-law refused to complete intercourse with Tamar, his brother's widow, and Yahweh killed him. Judah then promised his youngest son to Tamar, but as time passed he did nothing to fulfill his promise.

Meanwhile Judah's wife had died. Tamar resorted to extreme measures. She dressed as a whore and with her face covered enticed Judah into sexual relations with her. She became pregnant by her father-in-law. Although this act was not strictly in conformity with the levirate law, it was ultimately acceptable. She bore twin sons to carry on her husband's name.

According to the synoptic Gospels, the Sadducees presented Jesus with a problem related to levirate marriage. These particular Jews had no belief in the afterlife or in the resurrection, but they knew that Jesus, like the Pharisees and other religious Jewish groups, did believe in a heaven and a hell and in the resurrection. They posed a question: There were seven brothers. The first took a wife and died and left no children. The second took her and died without offspring. Then the third, and ultimately the seventh, and there were no children. Finally the woman died. In the resurrection, they asked, "Whose wife will she be for the seven who had her as wife?" Jesus responded that "when they rise from the dead, they neither marry nor are they given in marriage, but they are like angels in heaven" (Mark 12: 18–27 and parallels). According to Jesus there are no sexual relationships in heaven!

The biblical laws pertaining to incest do not seem to come into the picture when marriage between family members fulfills levirate rulings. Incest regulations apply in all other settings. Nor is the levirate marriage recognized as a form of polygamy, for the woman does not have more than one husband at a time.

4

Polygamy

Most men in biblical times had only one wife, but there were some who had more. Just when and how polygamy originated and developed is not known for sure. Some have pointed to Lamech, a descendant of Cain, who is the first person mentioned in the Bible with more than one wife (Gen. 4:19). Lamech is portrayed as an angry person who repaid any harm done to his group with vendetta justice. The argument is that polygamy began with a violent person. But Lamech is a fictional character and the legend associated with him is designed to explain the origins of music and the work of the smith.

The emphasis in the Bible on the importance of the family, and particularly on producing sons, may have been a contributing factor. When Sarah was barren, she gave her maid Hagar to Abraham as a second wife to produce offspring (Gen. 16:3). Jacob's two wives were sisters and, when Rachel was barren, she gave her slave girl Bilhah to Jacob (Gen. 30:1–4). Therefore the development of a large family and in particular the raising of sons was undoubtedly a factor in polygamous marriage.

When royalty married women from different cities and countries, the marriages helped to cement relationships between important powerful families and governments. King David married Jebusite women in Jerusalem after he had conquered that city, thus easing the transition from Jebusite to Hebrew leadership (2 Sam. 5:13). His son Solomon, whose harem was reputed to include "700 wives, princesses, and 300 concubines," appears to have been anxious to enter covenant relationships with groups everywhere in his area (1 Kings 11:1–3). In addition, there is some suggestion that in the case of a ruler, evidence of sexual vitality was an important asset. The fertility religions of the ancient Near East prized the sexual prowess of their various deities, and rituals were designed to obtain blessings from these life-giving divinities to enhance the increase of herds, flocks, and crops. A vital king was a symbol of a vital nation; a sexually active monarch symbolized an affinity with divine principles. The lust for power and the wish to retain power were clearly aspects of polygamy in royalty.

Sexual desire for a beautiful woman was what attracted David to Bathsheba (2 Sam. 11), and she was added to his harem. Love motivated Jacob in his wish to make Rachel his wife. He was tricked by her father, who substituted his older daughter Leah for Rachel on the wedding night. Jacob had already worked seven years to pay the required marriage price for Rachel; he then worked a second seven years for the woman he loved (Gen. 29:18–30).

Polygamous marriages were not necessarily happy marriages. Jealousy could be engendered if the husband appeared to prefer one woman more than another, as Rehoboam did in his love for Maacah (2 Chron. 11:21). Dissension arose when one woman was fertile and the other was not. Hagar looked down on Sarah, because Hagar provided a son for Abraham while Sarah was infertile (Gen. 16:4). Hannah was tormented by Peninnah, Elkanah's other wife, because Hannah had not given birth to a child (1 Sam. 1:16). It is not surprising that the Hebrew word for second wife, *tsarah*, comes from a root meaning "to distress" or "to vex" or "to feel rivalry." Whether conflicts arose when there were more than two wives cannot be known for certain. Within the larger harem, there would probably be some hierarchy with the oldest wife or the wife representing the most powerful family having more influence and status. The story of Esther, which is a Jewish story set in a Persian court, indicates that although one queen could be a favorite, the monarch could have a harem of beautiful women ready to satisfy his sexual needs. When Queen Vashti refused to conform to the king's wishes, he tapped his harem for a successor; and of course it was the beautiful Jewish woman Esther who became the king's favorite.

Polygamy is not widely practiced in the Western world. Among Muslims it is permissible for a man to have up to four wives at one time, but the practice is severely limited and is rapidly being outlawed. The Koranic statement about plural marriage is tied into a teaching on protecting orphans—a problem that may have been very significant in the warring days of early Islam. The teaching appears in Sura 4:3:

> Give the orphans their property and do not exchange the corrupt for the good; do not devour their property, certainly that is a great crime.
> If you fear that you will not act justly toward the orphans, marry such women as seem good to you—two, three, four; but if you fear that you will not deal equally, then only one.

The concept of equal treatment includes economic benefits and some sort of rotational pattern for sex. One woman is not to be preferred over another.

The Church of the Latter Day Saints, which developed in America during the nineteenth century and is now a worldwide religion popularly known as Mormonism, sanctioned polygamy in its early stages as not only natural but, for some, a preferred form of marriage. The doctrines of the church justified polygamy on the basis of Old Testament precedents. In a revelation received by the Mormon prophet and leader Joseph Smith in July 1843, reference was made to the concubines of Abraham and the patriarchs as well as to the wives and concubines of Moses, David, and Solomon. Smith was to be the restorer of the ancient order (*Doctrines and Covenant* 132:37–40). By the close of the century, Mormonism had come into conflict with the beliefs of other religions and with the United States government. Plural marriages were given up and Mormons conformed to the patterns found in the rest of American society.

There are still some few outposts of Mormon fundamentalists where individual males have several wives, but these groups lie outside of official Mormonism. Polygamy never became widespread in the Mormon communities, and by most estimates never exceeded 10 percent of Mormon families. Most polygamous families included the husband and two or three wives and children, or about seven members. The small size of the family is interesting because one of the intentions of polygamy was to create large families to accommodate the Mormon belief that there are in the universe a multitude of spirits waiting to be born. These spirits require corporeal bodies, and it was to help those spirits that large families were seen as desirable.

There were other factors that contributed to the abandonment of polygamy in Mormonism besides conflicts with other religious groups and the United States government. One was the problem of inheritance. Under civil law, only the first wife was recognized. Another revolved around temperamental factors, including the jealousy between women. A third was the economic hardships associated with plural marriages. In the pioneering days, several women about the home and farm could alleviate the burden of work falling upon a single wife. As the Mormon communities began to change, the support of many wives was not always an economic asset.

The polygamy issue was one of the divisive elements in the Mormon church. The Reorganized Church of the Latter Day Saints, which is an organization separate from the Church of the Latter Day Saints, disavowed polygamy from the start.

Polygamy, which means having more than one spouse at a time, has been virtually abandoned in the Western world. Perhaps it has been replaced by the newer pattern of sequential partners—a system in which couples marry, divorce, then marry other spouses, divorce, and so on, ad infinitum.

5

May-December Marriage

Marriages in which one spouse is considerably older than the other are popularly known as May–December marriages. They are often the subject of bawdy humor that reflects social uneasiness and often social prejudice. It is assumed that, if the older partner is male, he will be unable to sexually satisfy his wife and that she may begin to look for younger partners. If the woman is the older partner, the jokes will suggest that she ages in ways that make her physically ugly and perhaps sexually inept. There is cruelty in these characterizations, as there is cruelty in any humor that is designed to "put down" a particular group of people.

In biblical times, marriages between older men and younger women were not unusual, and they reflect the power and authority of the male in ancient Israel. There are no records of the marriage of older women to younger men. A man could have more than one wife at the same time; women were not permitted more than one husband at the same time. Women married young, but a male could marry at any age. Falling in love was not significant. The girl was a possession and under the authority of her father until he released her to another male, much in the way marriages are arranged in ultra-conservative Jewish families in Israel and in conservative Arab families throughout the Near East today.

After Sarah's death, Abraham married Keturah, who bore him six sons. In addition to Keturah, Abraham had concubines with whom he also copulated and who bore him children (Gen. 25:1 ff.). Scholars know that the Bible writers, keenly aware of linguistic affiliations, were seeking to trace the origins of various Semitic-speaking groups to Abraham (compare Gen. 25:12 ff.) and that the stories are pious fiction. But Abraham is also the model Jew. He is blessed beyond all others by his god Yahweh, and the blessings include longevity and virility.

How old was Abraham when he sired his second family? Sarah was 127 years old when she died (Gen. 23:1), and Abraham was ten years older than Sarah (Gen. 19:17). Abraham was therefore over 137 years old when he married Keturah, took concubines, and produced offspring. Because it was important that a woman was a virgin when she came to the marriage bed, one can assume that Keturah was young, perhaps in her teens, when she became Abraham's second wife. There is no suggestion that she may have been an older widow. The concubines selected by the patriarch would also be young women.

Marriages were arranged by male representatives of the family and in this case Abraham (or perhaps his servant) and Keturah's father or older brothers would arrange for the union. Abraham would pay a bride price (*mohar*) and Keturah would become his wife. There was no emphasis on "falling in love" as there is in Western culture. To the best of our knowledge such arrangements worked well in the ancient world and met the criteria for acceptable marriage. The purpose of the marriage was to produce offspring, and the woman's role was fulfilled when she bore children. There can be little doubt that the religious fiction surrounding Abraham was designed to teach the worshipers of Yahweh that in faithfulness to the religion and in loyalty to Yahweh there was a promise of rich benefits—long life, vital old age, and a large family.

Isaac, Abraham's son, was forty years old when he married. His bride, Rebekah, young and virginal, was in her teens. Such alliances were considered normal (Gen. 25:19 ff.). In the story that develops about the two sons of Isaac, Esau and Jacob, the manipulative role that Rebekah plays in the rivalry that grew up between the two brothers when Isaac was quite old demonstrates that she must have been considerably younger than her husband.

The story of Ruth's marriage to Boaz may also reflect a May–December marriage. When Ruth crept under Boaz's cloak as he slept on the threshing floor and laid herself down by his genitals ("feet"), he awoke and said to her: "May Yahweh bless you, my daughter, for you have made this last kindness greater than the first in that you have not gone after the young men whether rich or poor . . ." (Ruth 3:10). The term *daughter* may be a protective term or may indicate the age difference between Boaz and Ruth. His remark makes it clear that she was young enough to catch the attention of younger men. Her choice of Boaz was flattering to the older man. Ultimately she bore his child Obed, who was the grandfather of King David. The story is pious fiction and, although it may contain an accurate record of a part of David's genealogy, it appears to have been written for other purposes. It gives insight into the importance of the levirate-marriage custom and it is a counterthrust against Jews like Ezra and Nehemiah, who during the post-exilic period attacked marriages between Jews and non-Jews. This story points out that a marriage between a Moabite woman and a Hebrew produced the family of King David.

David's marriage to Bathsheba, which began as an adulterous affair, appears to have been a May–December marriage. When David first became involved with Bathsheba, he was in his forties or perhaps had reached the age of fifty. Bathsheba was young, the wife of one of David's warriors, and was possibly in her late teens. Despite the ugliness of the situation in which the relationship began, which included the murder of Uriah, Bathsheba's husband, the marriage seems to have worked well. The first child died, but the second child, Solomon, succeeded David to the throne after Bathsheba, Nathan, and Solomon successfully carried through a palace intrigue. Bathsheba seems to have been close to David when he was quite old, when he was perhaps becoming a bit senile. No other wife is mentioned at this stage of his life (1 Kings 1–2), despite the fact that David had taken some twenty other wives and concubines before Bathsheba. The attempt to help David prove himself sexually with Abishag, the Shunnamite beauty, failed—it was a May–December alliance that did not work out because David was impotent.

In our present society, May–December marriages are those that link two people who are separated in age by twenty or more years. The older partner may be anywhere between fifty years old and the mid-eighties; the younger from the late teens to the late thirties. Public attitudes toward these unions vary. Some condemn them as unseemly and seek pseudopsychological explanations to reenforce their disapproval. *She* (if she is younger) is seeking a father figure, or (if she is older) she is looking for a son. *He* (if he is older) is either a "dirty old man" or has a "daughter complex," or (if he is younger) he has a "mother complex." These popular "complexes" suggest that one is either marrying a parent or a child and that this can be interpreted as some subverted oedipus complex. The "dirty old man" (and "dirty old woman") label implies that there is something lecherous or lascivious in the relationship. There are also suggestions that the younger person marries the older for the money involved, or for "security," or because the younger person has something wrong with him/her and cannot "get" anyone younger, or because the younger person is enamored of power or wisdom or authority figures, and so on. The older person is trying to regain his/her youth, is seeking to deny aging, is after sleek young bodies, and so on.

Interestingly enough, those engaged in the relationship appear to be happy together and claim to love each other. May–December relationships have a low incidence of separation and divorce. It seems as though there is a very individualistic investment of personalities in such a relationship that separates it from marriages of people in the same age grouping. When Pablo Picasso married Jacqueline in 1954, she was twenty-eight, the divorced mother of a four-year-old. He was seventy-three and his personal life was in turmoil. When Picasso died in 1973 at the age of ninety-three, the love affair was still in full bloom. The paintings he created during the twenty-year love-affair with his wife are, according to critics, "messages of tenderness and passion." What did each partner bring to this union that made it so rich and beautiful? Other May–December couples comment on the depth of the love that unites them, on the potency of the relationship, and on the individualistic growth that blossoms in each partner. Much more study needs to be done in analyzing just what this special quality is.

Most often the public becomes aware of May–December marriages when one of the partners is a well-known person. May–December movie-star weddings, which extend from Charles Chaplin to Fred Astaire, capture public attention. Government officials (Strom Thurmond, for example) who marry younger partners are mentioned in the news and in national gossip magazines. The public follows the adventures of the couple, watching for every possible expression of affection or disaffection.

Most May–December marriages do not attract much public attention. They are between persons who are not prominent public figures. Their problems do not stem from the general public, but from family and acquaintances who do not approve. Parents may be very protective of their children and feel that somehow the marriage of one of their offspring to someone who is old enough to be a parent, or who may indeed be older than the parents, is not quite right. To what extent the oedipus patterns can be read into these feelings is not clear. Certainly fathers "fall in love with" their daughters, and mothers with their sons, and any man or woman who takes the child from the home is a threat to the established familial patterns. But when that person is as old as the parents, it becomes difficult to incorporate the new person into the family as "son" or "daughter."

Some of these feelings were dramatized in the warm comedy film *Harold and Maude*. Harold, a young man in his late teens falls in love with Maude, who is just about to turn eighty. The film makes it clear that they do have at least one sexual encounter that appears to satisfy and please both. Maude is much more realistic about the relationship than Harold, and she does "mother" him to some degree. But they enjoy each other. When Harold announces his decision to marry Maude, his mother reacts with horror and cannot accept the idea. The parish priest responds with disgust at the thought of Harold's firm young body being involved with the wrinkled and withered body of Maude. Neither seem to care about how Maude or Harold might feel about each other. This is often the attitude of parents and friends when those of different ages marry.

The independence of youth and the ability of young people to support themselves have relieved youth of the traditional dependency upon the family for support. It is not surprising to find young people from eighteen to twenty years old living in their own apartments, working at jobs they have found, caring for themselves, buying their own clothes, cooking their own food, and entertaining their own friends. They do not report to their parents when they come and go. They do not have to have their parents' approval of the friends they choose. They can sleep at a friend's house or have a friend sleep with them as they choose. However, when they find an older person whom they wish to marry, family disapproval can become a tremendous burden. Often they are faced with loss of family. The parents and relatives refuse to recognize the older partner. Family gatherings at which married brothers and sisters who found mates within their own age range are welcomed limit the welcome to the younger or older family member. The odd couple is isolated. There are genuine feelings of loss and of guilt for having failed to please the family.

Some clergy are open to such marriages. They will perform the ceremonies as they would officiate at the marriage of any other church member. Some, however, disapprove. They feel that there is something unnatural about the union. They see people as members of age groupings—a pattern that is echoed in church structure with youth groups, young married couples, singles groups, older married couples, senior citizens, and widows groups. There is a conviction that people of the same age group have a common heritage that binds them together and that separates them from those in other age groupings. Very little constructive help can come from those with such convictions.

Some therapists are also bound by theories that echo the church patterns. They believe there must be something not quite normal (but not really abnormal) prompting a young person to seek an older companion, particularly when the older person is of the younger partner's parents' age. They prefer not to deal with the pain of separation from the family that is troubling one or the other of the union but, instead, focus on what motivated these two people to come together. Why did the younger person "seek out" the older? Why did the older person "seek out" this very young adult? Why did each not find someone in their own age group? There is an implication that one or the other was *looking* for a partner in a different age bracket. Such therapists have little to offer and, indeed, they often succeed in adding new problems of insecurity to the already burdened couple.

On the other hand, there are therapists and clergy and families that seek the best for the two persons in love. They give aid and strength in helping each toward personal self-realization, toward helping to develop life patterns that strengthen and enhance the relationship, and offer support and encouragement toward a successful future. The Bible plays a very small role in this kind of union. Some who would use the Bible ignore the fact that, in the Bible, age (particularly the age of the male) appears to be irrelevant.

6

May-October Marriage

Not all marriages with notable differences in the ages of the participants can be labeled May–December. Many more marriages are between spouses who are separated by anywhere from five to twenty years. What is more significant is that now the older person is more likely than ever before to be the woman. As in the May–December alliances, these women are violating what society has come to expect is normal: that a woman will marry a man who is a few years her senior. We are calling such alliances May–October marriages.

We are in a new age initiated by the sixties, with its laid-back attitude toward age differences and its emphasis on the validity of individual human personality, and augmented by the seventies, with its efforts to liberate women. Views of sex have changed, and men and women have grown up and away from their high school concerns about whether the girl was six months older or ahead by one grade. Attitudes toward the role of men as participants in developing a home rather than as sole providers for the home have been relaxed. In one family the woman is six years older. She is an excellent business person with investment skills honed fine by experience and wisdom. Her twenty-two-year-old partner is happy to be at home with their two-year-old infant, to be the in-house parent, to care for the property, to prepare the meals and do the grocery shopping and the laundry. He is happy in his role, and she is delighted with the arrangement. They love each other passionately, enjoy each other's company, and really do not care what the outside world thinks of the arrangement, for they are accepted by family and friends.

In other families, both partners work and both contribute to maintaining a home. He is thirty and she is forty-four. Her children by a previous marriage are now on their own, his daughter is ten and lives part of the time with her mother and part of the time with her father and his older wife. They are happy together and the future has promise.

There are any number of marriages between couples where the male is older by ten or fifteen years. Young women in college complain that the males in their age group are still mentally, emotionally, and socially in junior high school, still trying ''to score'' for the sake of scoring. The older male is mature, is (it is hoped) past the scoring stage, and is interested in building a relationship that has both depth and meaning. They court the younger women and marry them.

There are those, including therapists and clergy, who look on such marriages with considerable skepticism. They use terms like *infatuation, buying younger companionship, the gigolo marriage, Mommy fixations, security blanket,* and so on. Couples involved in the relationship are often offended and argue that there is so much insecurity and impermanence in human relationships anyway that these well-meaning advisors are actually detractors who may contribute to future dissension by sowing seeds of doubt or insecurity. They seek pastors who will help them to enhance their relationships and who will bring the blessing of the faith. They wish for therapists who will help them work at their marriage by aiding them to develop the attitudes and patterns of life that will strengthen the union.

But there are built-in problems that need recognition. Older women fear the onset of age marked by flabby thighs, sagging breasts, wrinkles, and stretch marks. They no longer purchase bikini swimsuits. The older man watches his softening belt line, the graying hair, the development of wrinkles. No matter how much the partner may praise these features as beautifully mature lines, there is the constant awareness of one person approaching old age more closely than the other. Much can be done through diet, exercise, and the miracles of skin care, but the years continue to accumulate and the calendar cannot be denied.

Society adds to the dis-ease. While friends and associates will accept the couple as a couple, there is always the moment when an indiscreet guest at a party comments on the beauty of "your daughter" or the graciousness of "your son." Good humor and relaxation in the relationship together with clear evidence of the commitment of the couple to each other can get the two past these situations.

More serious problems develop over the matter of children: They had been married four years. He was thirty and she was forty-two. Her daughters were nineteen and twenty years old and living in their own apartments. He wanted children and she agreed. She became pregnant and after three months suffered a miscarriage. She was devastated. He was angry and implied that she might be getting too old to bear. The result was a painful divorce during which she was made to feel aged, discarded, and unworthy of her young, athletic husband.

There is good biblical precedence for the older man–younger woman marriage. Isaac and Rebecca were separated by at least twenty years, and Boaz was notably older than Ruth. With the liberation of women, the privileges that have traditionally been given to men should now become theirs too. Magazine advertisements show the man with graying hair surrounded by young women fawning over him because he uses some after-shave lotion or other product. Similar advertisements might portray young men being drawn to older women. Whatever it will take to change public attitude needs exploration. One might wish that the traditional religious organizations that look to the Bible for guidance in faith and behavior might become leaders by welcoming and doing whatever they can to strengthen the growing number of May–October relationships.

7

Marriage to an "Outsider"

On July 1, 1982, 4,148 followers of the Reverend Sun Myung Moon were married in a mass ceremony held in Madison Square Garden in New York City. The majority of the American members were being united to young people from other countries, including Korea and Japan. The choice of mates was made by the church. The mixing of races was in accord with the teachings of the Reverend Moon, who believes that such unions will hasten the unification of humankind. The fact that the young couples could not (in some cases) communicate in words with one another was irrelevant for the moment—they would learn. The marriages were part of the steps necessary for salvation; they were in fulfillment of a religious duty. Love for one another in the romantic sense was not important; what was important was the theological conviction that each was involved in a divine destiny that would affect the world.

For many Westerners, the ceremony was a violation of the American dream of finding and falling in love with the perfect mate and of living together, working together, building a family together, not for the benefit of humankind, but for self-fulfillment. There was no American "honeymoon" for the Moonie new-lyweds; indeed, cohabitation and sexual unions would come only when the Reverend Moon, the "true father," decided that it was the proper time. These young people are "different." They have joined a movement that has an Eastern origin, that is determined to break the barriers that separate races, but at the same time a movement whose members are subject to the wishes of the messiah figure of the Reverend Sun Myung Moon.

Biblical Marriage to Foreigners

Marriages between Hebrews and those of different national or ethnic backgrounds or who were worshipers of gods other than Yahweh did take place. But such unions are discouraged in most biblical writings. Abraham worried that his son Isaac might marry a Canaanite woman. He sent his servant to the family of Nahor, Abraham's brother, to find a suitable wife. Isaac married his cousin Rebekah, who was chosen by the servant as the proper young woman for his master's son. Rebekah went to join her fiance without having seen him, and when she did meet Isaac she kept him from seeing her by remaining veiled (Gen. 24). After the marriage agreements had been completed, he took her to his tent, where the marriage was physically consummated.

Rebekah worried lest her son Jacob marry a Hittite woman. She sent him to his uncle Laban, where he married two of his cousins, Leah and Rachel (Gen. 27:46–29:30). These stories present patriarchal role models for Jewish marriages. Just as the founders of the faith took precautions against intermarriage, so must each Jew protect the heritage by marrying within the faith.

Not every Hebrew adhered to these customs. Esau married a Canaanite (Gen. 36:2). Joseph married a foreign woman (Gen. 41:45), and so did Moses (Exod. 2:21). When Samson expressed his desire for a Philistine woman, his parents protested but to no avail (Judg. 14). These few examples of intermarriage by hero figures probably represent a sampling of what was a much wider practice.

The greatest violator of the doctrine of marriage within the group was Solomon. Although the Deuteronomic editors who compiled the records during the early part of the sixth century B.C.E. could state that "Solomon loved Yahweh" (1 Kings 3:3), they could also note that he violated Yahweh's regulations:

Now King Solomon loved many alien women: Pharaoh's daughter, Moabite, Ammonite, Edomite, Sidonian, Hittite women from the peoples concerning whom Yahweh had said to the Israelites: You shall not have coitus with them and they shall not have coitus with you, lest they turn your hearts towards their gods; Solomon was joined to them in love. And he had seven hundred wives, princesses, and three hundred concubines, and his wives turned his heart away. And it happened, in Solomon's old age, that his wives turned his heart [mind] after other gods, and his heart was not at peace with Yahweh his god as was the heart of his father David. [1 Kings 11:1–6]

The account reports that Solomon built shrines for these alien deities and actively participated in their worship rites. It is for such apostasy rather than for the number of wives and concubines that the king was condemned.

Solomon's marriages had political and social significance. Politically, they linked the Hebrew court to prominent families in Canaan and to the royal courts and prominent families in surrounding nations. Socially, the numerous wives and concubines testified to the king's virility, a significant factor for the welfare of the nation. A virile king symbolized a virile people. The editors made Solomon an example of the danger of falling away from the national religion that resulted from the marriages to foreign women.

In the post-exilic period (fifth century B.C.E.), Nehemiah and Ezra took up the issue of intermarriage with new vigor. Nehemiah required an oath from the people of Jerusalem that they would not give their daughters in marriage to foreigners and would not take foreign wives for their sons (Neh. 10:30). He had learned that intermarriage bastardized the Hebrew language and weakened the faith (Neh. 13:23 ff.). Ezra went further in his demand for reform. He required that foreign wives be divorced (Ezra 10:11). Most scholars believe that the story of Ruth was composed about this same time as a counterargument to the demands of Nehemiah and Ezra. Ruth, a Moabitess, married Boaz, a Hebrew, and this couple became the progenitors of King David. If the most famous king of Israel could come from such a union, intermarriage could not be all bad!

Warnings about the danger of association with strange (alien) women occur in the book of Proverbs (2:16; 5:3–22, etc.). For some reason, foreign women appear to have exercised a strange fascination for Hebrew youth and were therefore a threat to their morals.

The early Christians also sought to protect the purity of the faith. The apostle Paul prohibited marriage with unbelievers. In a brief note in what is now 2 Corinthians, he wrote:

> Do not be mismated with unbelievers. What is the relationship between righteousness and wickedness? What fellowship can light have with darkness? What accord has Christ with Belial [Satan]? What does a believer share with an unbeliever? What agreement has God's temple with idols? And we are the temple of the living God. [2 Cor. 6:14–16]

Paul reinforced his statements with a series of quotations from Jewish scripture, including a command which he interpreted to mean that Christians should be separated from unbelievers. If a Christian was married to a nonbeliever and that nonbeliever was willing to remain married, Paul believed that the marriage relationship should continue.

> For the non-believing husband is consecrated through his believing wife and the non-believing wife is consecrated through her believing husband. Otherwise your children would be unclean, but as it is they are holy. If the unbeliever wishes to separate, let it be done; the believing husband or wife is not bound in such a circumstance . . . Wife, how do you know that you will not save your husband? Husband, how do you know that you will not save your wife? [1 Cor. 7:12–16]

Later, the writer of 1 Peter 3:1–2 advised the wife to show patience, chastity, and reverence so that she might convert her husband to the Christian faith.

The early Christian teachings reflect the idea of a superior faith that set believers apart from unbelievers, who could do little but pollute the purity of the believer. The mystical embracing of the unbeliever suggested by Paul implies that whether the nonbeliever likes it or not she/he is included in the faith by some sort of spiritual osmosis.

The importance of marrying within the faith system is still stressed. Most rabbis, ministers, and priests refuse to officiate at interfaith weddings unless the partner outside of the faith takes instruction and goes through some sort of conversion rite and, in some cases, agrees to raise any children in the faith. The fears associated with intermarriage have not faded in Jewish and Christian communities. Intermarriage tends to weaken familial religious patterns and hence weakens the community of faith. Intermarriage represents the mixing of the true believer's thinking with ideas that are pagan or that may represent some distortion of what is conceived to be the "truth." Such a union, in religious parlance, would not be blessed by God. The fears expressed are for the strength of the faith, for the faith of the true believer, and for the faith in which the children will be raised. Most liberal Protestant clergy will perform weddings for couples coming from differing branches of the Protestant church. Depending on the gulf that separates the two denominations, religious instruction and advisement may be necessary. Most conservative Christians insist that both join the "true faith." Roman Catholic clergy do not marry couples where one member persists in remaining a Jew or an atheist or a Protestant. Jewish clergy, with few exceptions, will not marry a Jew to a non-Jew.

The problem of racial intermarriage has lessened to some degree in large cities, but remains a troublesome issue in smaller towns and those with conservative clergy. Men in the military brought back wives from Korea and Vietnam and Japan. Black–oriental marriages and black–white marriages became more common with the rise of black consciousness. As housing restrictions were abandoned and school integration became standard, children and adults with differing racial, national, ethnic, and religious backgrounds found themselves in the same social situations, supporting some of the same causes. By the time the children reached college, many had friends from these varied groups, and intermarriage seemed a natural consequence.

But old prejudices die slowly. Parental concern about the physical appearances of the children of interracial unions (many are very beautiful), societal disgust over a black kissing an oriental or an oriental engaging in sexual intercourse with a white is still prevalent. Some clergy discourage interracial marriages with the same passion that they refuse to perform interfaith marriages. Despite the fact that the couple belong to the same denomination, the clergy point out that the children will have social problems in adjusting to a furcated society. Paul could write of the oneness in the faith in Christ where there were neither slaves nor free persons, Jew nor non-Jew (Gal. 3:28), but racial and religious bigotry are still rampant among conservative religious groups.

Many young people having been rejected by their own religious groups seek out local justices of the peace or turn to humanistic religious organizations like the Ethical Culture Societies of the American Ethical Union for guidance, for insight, and for an officiant for the marriage. Leaders in these groups do not demand adherence to a particular faith system or the acceptance of religious dogma from the couple. They respond to the need for help in giving social acceptance to the statement of love that two people wish to make to each other. Nor do they actively seek to proselytize; their emphasis is on human well-being rather than on the winning of converts.

8

Surrogate Parents

Surrogate Mothers

In biblical times, when a married woman failed to conceive, it was believed that nonconception was due to the deity closing the womb. In such circumstances she might provide her husband with her personal slave who would bear the child for her. It is possible that the pregnant woman would sit on her mistress's lap, and the child would emerge from the vagina and be received through the legs of her mistress, who could then, in a sense, claim the child as her own.

When Rachel failed to produce children for her husband, Jacob, she was angry and demanded that he give her children lest she die. He responded that he could not do what only the deity could do. Rachel then said: "Here is my servant Bilhah; copulate with her that she may give birth on my knees and I will have children through her" (Gen. 30). Jacob had sexual intercourse with Bilhah, and when a son who was called Dan was born, Rachel claimed that the deity had given her a son. Leah, having passed menopause, also gave Jacob a slave woman, named Zilpah, who bore children for her mistress. The arrangement, which may seem to be a bit strange in the twentieth century, appears to have been a perfectly acceptable one in most cases. When Sarah did not bear a child for Abraham, she gave him her slave Hagar, and the child born was called Ishmael. The relationship between Hagar and Sarah was anything but pleasant, and there is no evidence to suggest that Sarah ever accepted Ishmael as her own child produced through a surrogate mother.

Surrogate mothers have come into the news once again. In 1980, a thirty-seven-year-old Illinois woman who used the pseudonym Elizabeth Kane to mask her real identity announced that she was bearing a child for a couple who lived in Kentucky. The wife of the couple had a blocked fallopian tube and could not have a child. Kane was inseminated clinically with the husband's sperm. Kane, who is a happily married mother of three children of her own, insisted she was acting out of love, but the fact that she was paid between $8,000 and $10,000 for her services prompted some news writers to derisively refer to the "rent-a-womb business."

Since Kane made the case public, the cost of surrogate mothering has apparently doubled.

It is estimated that at present (1983) there are approximately fifty children in America who were born of surrogate mothers, and Los Angeles attorney William Handel has stated publicly that he has helped childless couples find women willing to serve as surrogate mothers.

The development is not without its problems. In 1981 a woman who had agreed to become a surrogate mother decided she wanted to keep the child. The sperm donor and his wife sued for custody, but it was ruled by a California judge that the "natural mother" could keep the child. Most states have laws prohibiting any form of baby buying, and there are some legal authorities who are asking if paying a surrogate mother might not be the equivalent of purchasing an infant. In other states legislation is being considered that would legalize the payment of money to a surrogate mother for her services.

In addition to childless couples who might wish to employ a surrogate mother, there are others who are attracted by the idea. There are males who would like to have their own child to raise but who do not want to get married. They would donate the sperm, the surrogate mother would be artificially inseminated, and the child would join the family of the father without ever knowing the mother who provided the ovum. Professional women who do not wish to go through pregnancy have expressed willingness to have their husbands donate sperm for surrogate mothers. The creation of sperm banks also provides for the possibility of surrogate fathers, men whose sperm would be used to artificially inseminate single women who wanted to bear their own children.

But questions have been raised. Some of them are related to the possible personal problems of adjustment that may arise later. Will the child's parents ever feel that they have done something not quite right in producing a child in this manner? Will the father feel that the child is more his than his wife's because his sperm was used and she really had no part in the whole scheme except to grant approval? Will the child's real mother even want to try to get in touch with the child? Will the woman who did not bear her son or daughter have problems in adjusting to a family that, in a sense, she has acquired by adoption? Will the child who is produced by sperm from a sperm bank ever try to find his or her real father? Should each pair of prospective parents be required to have extensive therapy before engaging a surrogate parent? What happens if the child is something less than a perfect infant?

A further development of the fertilization process includes the birth of so-called test-tube babies. The first such birth was announced in July 1978 with the birth in England of Louise Brown. Her mother, Lesley Brown, was unable to conceive naturally. An ovum was removed from her body and fertilized in a petri dish with the sperm of her husband John Brown. The fertilized ovum was then reintroduced into Lesley's womb, and she carried her child to successful birth. When Dr. Georgeanna Jones and her husband Dr. Howard Jones announced from

Eastern Virginia Medical School that they were successfully engaged in in-vitro (in-a-dish) fertilization of ova, they were accused of playing God because they discarded fertilized ova that were less than perfect. They froze the embryos for research, and their work was the initial step in what could become an assembly-line production of human beings.

One of the important theological issues is identical with one that is raised in the abortion controversy. Those who believe that humans possess an immortal soul disagree as to the exact moment the soul "enters" the human personality. For some, including most Roman Catholics, it is at the moment of conception, when the sperm penetrates the ovum. Thus to discard fertilized ova because they are imperfect is to destroy human life. Others, basing their argument on an interpretation of Genesis 2:7, which states that when the deity breathed into the nostrils of the man he had formed from clay, "man became a living being," would argue that the fertilized ovum, the developing human embryo, receives the "soul" when it begins to breathe and not until that moment. Of course the biblical text merely states that the deity animated the clay figurine, the man (*adam*) had been formed from earth (*adamah*), and it became a living creature (*nephesh*)—not a creature possessing a soul, but a creature that was alive and breathing. Animation of infants by blowing into their nostrils is also practiced by Arab midwives. The biblical narrative reflects a Near Eastern custom that has a long history that extends into the present. It really cannot be used to either support or reject the idea of the soul, although biblical exegesis will not inhibit those who wish to interpret the passage differently.

In actuality, the idea of a soul is a recent development in Jewish and Christian belief systems. The Sadducees, who were the priesthood in charge of the ancient Jewish temple, did not believe in a "soul" that existed apart from the human or that came into the human from outside. The individual was a psychosomatic unity that existed as long as it continued to breathe and that ceased to exist at death. Other people believed in the existence of souls, including the Egyptians and the Persian followers of Zarathustra, but not the Hebrew religionists. In biblical literature, belief in after-death existence develops just before the beginning of Christianity and can be found only in the book of Daniel in the Jewish scriptures. It was accepted from the beginning by the Christian belief system. There is no guidance given in Christian or Jewish scriptures about the time the soul became a part of the human. The arguments have developed outside of the Bible.

Surrogate Fathers

Surrogate fathers are those who donate sperm that can be used to fertilize women whose husbands are infertile. The donated sperm is frozen until it is needed. At that time it is unfrozen and introduced into the woman's vaginal tract or through the cervix into the uterus by a cooperating medical doctor or, in some cases, by the woman herself. One of the most publicized sperm banks is the Repository for Germinal Choice in Escondido, California, the so-called Nobel sperm bank, whose donors are all intelligent and accomplished men.

The sperm is supposed to be available only to married couples, but Dr. Afton Blake, a Los Angeles psychologist, obtained sperm and became pregnant despite the fact that she was single. The sperm of her first two donors did not "take," but with the sperm of the third donor she became pregnant. Her child, a boy, will never know his true father, although the organizers of the bank provided Dr. Blake with details about the donor's interests and what was known of his biological heredity.

The condemnations of this form of insemination have included the familiar "humans playing God" objections and questions about a child growing up in a society with this kind of family heritage—an anonymous father and the possibility of step-brothers and -sisters in abundance. Fears about the attempts to produce a super race have also surfaced. If the state could ever assume the responsibility for selective breeding, sex could be reduced to nothing more than pure pleasure and parenting would be designed to breed and raise superchildren.

The recipient of the sperm is always eager to believe that the child will inherit the best qualities of both parents. One cannot help but recall the wisdom attributed to George Bernard Shaw when Lady Astor proposed to him that they should have an offspring. "Just think," she is supposed to have said, "it could have your brains and my looks." To which Shaw replied, "Yes, but what if it had my looks and your brains?"

9

Circumcision

Circumcision is a form of sexual mutilation that involves the cutting away of part or all of the prepuce, which is the loose fold of skin that covers the glans, the head of the penis. The "cutting around," as the word signifies, has been practiced in various parts of the world as far back as we can trace human history.

In the ancient Near Eastern world, circumcision was practiced by the Egyptians, the Hebrews, and other Semites, but not by the Babylonians or the Assyrians. The Philistines who entered Palestine about the same time as the Hebrews did not practice circumcision and hence were referred to by the Hebrews as "the uncircumcised"—a term of contempt.

A relief from the Sixth Dynasty tomb of Ankh-ma-Hor at Sakkarah portrays the circumcision of two youths in what can only be understood as a puberty rite marking the coming into manhood. A mortuary priest squats on his haunches before one standing youth whose hands are firmly held by an adult assistant. The priest holds the boy's penis in his left hand and in the right hand has a circular flint with which he is removing the prepuce. He says to the assistant, "Hold him, do not let him faint," and the assistant responds, "I will do as you request." The other youth being circumcised is also standing before the squatting priest. He has placed his left hand on the priest's head, as if to steady himself, his right hand is by his side. He says to the priest, "Thoroughly remove [rub off] what is there." The priest replies, "I will cause it to heal." The priest holds the penis in his left hand and in his right hand is a large flint knife with which he is cutting off the foreskin.[1]

The significance of circumcision for the Egyptians is not known. Herodotus, who visited Egypt in the fifth century B.C.E., reported that "they practice circumcision for the sake of cleanliness, for they place cleanliness before propriety . . ." (II, 37). A mythological reference in Chapter 17 of the Book of the Dead states that the sun-god Ra circumcised himself and that from the drops of blood two protective deities came into being, so that perhaps there is a prophylactic symbolism in the Egyptian ritual. However, not all Egyptians were circumcised. X-rays of the mummy of the Pharaoh Ahmose (Eighteenth Dynasty, sixteenth century B.C.E.)

demonstrate that he was not circumcised, and it is possible that his successor Amenhotep I also was uncircumcised.[2]

The Hebrew rite of circumcision appears to have had a long history, for there are two references to the use of flint knives. The first is in a folk tale associated with Moses in the wilderness:

> Then it happened, at a stopping place along the way, that Yahweh met him [Moses] and tried to kill him. Then Zipporah [Moses' Midianite wife] took a piece of flint and cut off her son's foreskin and touched his feet [genitals] with it, saying, "You are a blood-bridegroom to me." So he let him alone. At that time she said "blood-bridegroom" in reference to circumcision. [Exod. 4:24–26]

The textual and interpretation problems associated with this brief passage are extensive and will not be developed here.[3] It is not clear why Yahweh wanted to kill his chosen deliverer. It is clear that the circumcision had apotropaic implications, for Yahweh did not kill Moses. Presumably the blood of the foreskin was wiped upon Moses' genitals, although the text does not make that clear. The saying "you are a blood-bridegroom to me," appears to have had some social or cultural significance in the circumcision rite that we do not now understand. Nor is it clear why Zipporah performed the circumcision rather than Moses.

The use of a flint suggests a pre-iron age (before the twelfth century B.C.E.) history, although the use of flint could be explained in two ways. First, flint chips, which can be razor sharp, are easily accessible so that Zipporah used what was at hand. Second, the rite has its roots in Egypt, where flint knives seem to have been used.

The second reference to a flint-cutting tool for circumcision occurs in Joshua 5:2–3 and forms part of the seventh-century collection of legends associated with the Hebrew invasion of Palestine.

> At that time, Yahweh said to Joshua, "Get for yourselves flint knives and sit down to circumcise the people of Israel for a second time. So Joshua made flint knives and circumcised the people of Israel on the hill of foreskins.

The legend goes on to explain that the reason the Hebrews had not been circumcised earlier was because they had been in the desert for forty years and did not listen to Yahweh's commands. The only way they could enter "the promised land" was by being made acceptable to the deity by circumcision. The legend also explains a spot called "the hill of foreskins" and attributes the name of nearby Gilgal to the belief that through this act of cutting the "reproach of Egypt" was "rolled away" (from the root *gll* "to roll over"). Actually the term *gilgal* means a "circle of stones," but the writer employed a play on sound to give it a new meaning.

The text is not as clear as one would wish. Most scholars follow the Greek (LXX) version and used the words "sit down to" (as we have done) rather than the

Masoretic (Hebrew) text, which reads "begin again to." The squatting posture of the Egyptian priests immediately comes to mind. The use of flint goes back to antiquity, but may also indicate the presence of flint shards in the area.

A much later tradition, added to the biblical narratives during the post-exilic period (after the sixth century B.C.E.), links circumcision to Abraham. According to this legend, the deity made a covenant with Abraham, promising that a host of nations would be sired by the patriarch. For their part of the covenant, Abraham and his offspring would be loyal followers of their god. Just as symbols were used to mark human agreements, circumcision became the mark of this new covenant. The account that appears in Genesis 17 is summarized in a few verses. Abraham was told:

> . . . on your part, you must keep my covenant, you and your descendants . . . every male among you must be circumcised. You shall cut off the flesh of your foreskin, and that will be the symbol of the covenant between us. Throughout all your generations every male shall be circumcised at the age of eight days . . . [Gen. 17:10–12]

The demand also pertained to all slaves, including those from foreign countries. The agreement ends by warning that any uncircumcised male must be excommunicated from his people, because noncircumcision was tantamount to a broken convenant. This legend, like other religious fiction, answered what must have been a basic question: "Why do we circumcise?" The answer was: "Because it is a symbol of our agreement with our deity." Without circumcision one could not belong to the divinely ordained family of Israel. Because circumcision was performed upon infants, it was removed from what may have been its earlier significance—the coming into manhood or preparation for marriage—and became a symbol of Judaism.

When the Hivites of Shechem wished to marry into one of the clans associated with the partriarch Jacob (the Dinah group), they were required to undergo circumcision (Gen. 34). When they were in the uncomfortable state of healing, they were slaughtered by the Hebrews.

David wished to marry Saul's daughter Michal. The bride-payment (*mohar*) for a king's daughter would ordinarily be beyond the resources of a soldier, even one who was close to the royal family. Saul, who by this time was envious of and suspicious of David, saw an opportunity to rid himself of this young upstart. He requested as *mohar* 100 Philistine foreskins, assuming accurately one might imagine that the Philistine males would not yield their prepuces without battle. David overpaid with 200 foreskins, thus increasing Saul's hostility toward him, even while giving his daughter to be David's bride (1 Sam. 18:17–29). The circumcision of the Philistines did not transform them into Hebrews; one would assume that David killed them in order to circumcise them.

Circumcision was used as a symbol of conversion to Judaism. During the Babylonian exile of the Jews, the people of Edom moved into southern Judea and established themselves around Hebron. About 120 B.C.E., John Hyrcanus conquered this area for the Jews and compelled the Idumeans to be circumcised and to obey Jewish law if they wished to remain in the area. The story is told by the Jewish historian Josephus (*Antiquities* XIII. ix.1) and perhaps indicates why the Jews in Jesus' time never really accepted King Herod. He was a Jew, but an Idumean Jew, a half-Jew, so to speak—one who came in by forced conversion.

Some Jews attempted to remove the sign of circumcision. When the Greek rulers who succeeded Alexander the Great divided his kingdom among themselves, Palestine was a buffer state between Egypt and Syria. From both countries Greek influence impacted upon Jewish culture and many young Jews decided they preferred the Greek way of life to the Jewish. They began to wear Greek clothing, eat Greek (nonkosher) food, and exercise in the Greek gymnasium, where they would be seen in the nude. Their lack of a prepuce was an embarrassment, and some underwent operations to hide the mark of circumcision (1 Maccabees 1:15: Josephus, *Antiquities* XII. v.1). This would be done by pulling the skin of the penis forward and forming at least a partial prepuce. When Antiochus IV persecuted the Jews during this same period, he added insult to injury by forbidding the circumcision of male infants (1 Macc. 1:60 f; 2 Macc. 6:10).

At first the cutting was performed by the father and was therefore a family ritual. Abraham circumcised Isaac when the infant was eight days old (Gen. 21:4), but Ishmael, his son by Hagar, was thirteen when circumcised (Gen. 17:25). Later this ritual was performed by specialists. The apostle Paul states that he was circumcised on the eighth day (Phil. 3:5) and Jesus was, too (Luke 2:21).

The first Christian missionaries to move out of Palestine into the Mediterranean world were Jews who had become Christians. They would go to the Jewish synagogue in a given city and begin to preach that Jesus was the Jewish Messiah. (Compare Acts 13:14; 14:1; etc.) The congregation might include a number of Greeks who were drawn to Judaism because it was monotheistic and had a code of conduct but who would not become Jews because they did not want to confine their diet to kosher food and did not want to be circumcised. At first there was a split within the early Christian community. There were those who argued that one must become a Jew before becoming a Christian and that that included circumcision. Against this circumcision, the apostle Paul and others who agreed with him argued that, in the Christian faith, circumcision was unnecessary (Acts 15). In a letter written to Christians in Galatia, Paul argues that those who want circumcision do it so that "they can glory in your flesh" (Gal. 6:12). So furious does he become with his opponents that he writes that he wishes that the members of the circumcision party ". . . those who unsettle you would castrate themselves" (Gal. 5:12).

Paul was engaged in a transformation of the meaning of circumcision. Just as the prophet Jeremiah in the seventh century B.C.E. had called for a new circumcision of the heart signifying a commitment of intent to follow Yahweh and suggesting that simply the cutting of the flesh did not put one in league with the deity (Jer. 9:25 f.), so Paul claimed that in Jesus as the Christ something new had evolved that went beyond circumcision to bind Christians in a new covenantal fellowship that disregarded human marks of separation, including race (Jew vs. Greek), circumcision (vs. noncircumcision), slave (vs. free man), and so on (Col. 3:10–11). He warns the Philippian congregation to be on guard against the flesh-cutters (Phil. 3:2) but points out to the followers in Corinth that they should not put undue emphasis on circumcision. If they were circumcised, not to attempt to cover the scars; if they were not, to remain uncircumcised. The matter was really unimportant to the faith. What mattered was the inner commitment to the new faith (Rom. 2:29, etc.).

Circumcision in the Modern World

Circumcision is widely practiced in different parts of the world. In a few remote places, ancient practices remain. For example, the rite of circumcision among the Kisii of Nigeria is reminiscent of ancient Egyptian customs. The adolescent boy about to become a man stands naked before a tree. His hands are raised above his head to clasp the trunk of the tree behind him. He looks steadfastly ahead as though fixing his eyes on some distant spot and as if he has numbed himself to pain. Two family members stand beside him, one with a spear, the other with a club, both threatening violence if he should give any sign of pain. The circumciser, who has been wined and dined by the family and who may be slightly drunk, squats before the boy, just as the Egyptian priest squatted before the youths in the Sakkara scene. He pulls the penis by the foreskin and with a knife circles the glans and from the bleeding phallus removes the foreskin. The raw and still bleeding penis is packed with herbs and one hopes it will heal without infection. There are, of course, certain songs and rituals, but the center of the ceremony is the removal of the foreskin and the boy's coming into manhood.[4]

Circumcision is widely practiced in the modern Western world. It is usually performed in a hospital by doctors with the consent of the parents. In other words, the person who is circumcised has no voice in the decision-making process. Just why circumcision is performed is not really clear. Those with Jewish background, even though they have abandoned their traditional faith and customs, have it done, perhaps to keep the parents happy or because it has been a family or ethnic tradition or for reasons of cleanliness (even though there is no reason for a noncircumcised individual not to be as clean as a circumcised one). Some will cite theories that state there is less likely to be cancer of the cervix among women whose husbands are circumcised—a claim that lacks evidence.

Non-Jews have their sons circumcised for some of these same reasons— cleanliness, prevention of cancer of the cervix, and of course because Jesus and the early Christians were circumcised. Many simply go along with their doctors, who tend to be medical traditionalists.

There are, however, a number of young married couples who question this traditional mutilation of the flesh. They have decided to wait until their sons are old enough to decide for themselves whether they wish to have the prepuce removed. They avoid the arguments over whether a circumcised penis is more or less aesthetically pleasing than one that is not circumcised, arguing that beauty is in the eye of the beholder. They are familiar with the findings in sex research that have demonstrated that a circumcised penis is just as sensitive as an uncircumcised one and that the problem of premature ejaculation is not related to the operation. They refuse to let the Bible and biblical traditions affect their judgment. They are prepared to teach their children proper habits of bodily cleanliness as matters of personal health. Nor are they moved by the argument that circumcision may remove castration fears, because, in a sense, the mutilation has already been done.

Female Circumcision

Some cultures have practiced mutilation of the genitals of females. Sometimes the inner labia and the clitoris are completely removed. Sometimes the clitoris is burned out with rock salt or is extended and cut off. The intention is to diminish the woman's pleasure in sex and to help ensure her fidelity to her husband. Fortunately this barbarous custom is becoming extinct in many parts of the world.[5]

A minor operation is sometimes performed on women to clear adhesions that might interfere with sexual response. These adhesions result from the accumulation of smegma secreted under the "hood," or prepuce, of the clitoris.

NOTES

1. For a picture of the scene, see James B. Pritchard, ed., *The Ancient Near East in Pictures* (*ANEP*) (Princeton, 1969), No. 629. For a translation of the text, see that of John A. Wilson in James B. Pritchard, ed., *Ancient Near Eastern Texts Relating to the Old Testament (ANET)* (Princeton, 1950), p. 326, footnote 2.

2. James E. Harris and Kent R. Weeks, *X-raying the Pharaohs* (New York, 1973), pp. 126f., 130.

3. See Brevard S. Childs, *The Book of Exodus* (Philadelphia, 1974), pp. 90–104.

4. I am grateful to Arthur Dobrin, Leader of the Ethical Society of Long Island, for the information about the Kisii ritual.

5. It is still practiced by some tribes in upper Egypt, in Arabia, and in Oman. See Wendell Phillips, *Unknown Oman* (New York, 1966).

10

Testicles

Although the penis could be mutilated by circumcision, the testicles were to be protected. Apparently they were recognized as the source of the life-producing fluid, although the Hebrews would have no way of distinguishing between sperm and seminal fluid. Somewhere in their evolution, the Hebrews learned what their neighbors in nearby countries had also learned, that without testicles a man (or animal) could not produce offspring. They would know also that a man without testicles could still engage in sexual intercourse.

The eunuch was one whose testicles had been removed or damaged or crushed, and such men were often court officials in the ancient world. Potiphar, a eunuch in the Egyptian court, was married (Gen. 39). Though he would never produce offspring he could still enjoy the benefits of married life and could, perhaps, engage in sex and satisfy his wife's needs. In Persia, eunuchs were in charge of the royal harem (Esther 2:3). Should they dare to engage in sexual intercourse with any of the harem women, the monarch knew that they would not impregnate the women; the children of the harem would be the children of the king.

Hebrew kings collected taxes to support palace eunuchs (1 Sam 8:15; 1 Kings 22:9; Jer. 38:7). If the eunuchs were used by their masters for sodomy, it is not recorded.

Eunuchs were not considered the equals of Hebrews with undamaged testicles. They could not, according to Deuteronomic law, participate in temple ritual (Deut. 23:1), and a eunuch could not become a priest. Eunuchs were in a category like those who had an infectious disease or an imperfect body, for none of these could serve Yahweh as priests (Lev. 21:20). So fastidious were the Hebrew lawmakers about perfection in the presence of the deity that a castrated animal was considered to be unsuitable for a sacrificial offering (Lev. 22:24).

The testicles were the seat of the male generative power and had to be protected at all costs. If there was a street brawl between two men and the wife of one man reached out to help her husband by seizing his opponent's testicles, she was punished by mutilation—her hand was cut off (Deut. 25:11–12). Oaths were taken on the testicles. When Abraham sent his servant to find a suitable wife for Isaac, the old man had Eleazer put his hand under his (Abraham's) thigh and swear on his testicles to fulfil his mission (Gen. 24:2 f.). When Joseph's father was dying, he asked his son to put his hand beneath his thigh and swear on his testicles that he would be buried in the family tomb (Gen. 47:29). There is no condemnation of one man touching the sexual organs of another, nor is there any reference to uncovering "nakedness." Oath-taking was not considered a sexual gesture.

A sixth-century prophet whose writings were added to the book of Isaiah stated that the eunuch would be admitted to the court of Yahweh (Isaiah 56:3), but there is no evidence that his teachings were ever heeded by the Jews. An Ethiopian eunuch was admitted to the Christian community, but no temple rituals were involved and no sacred precincts could be violated (Acts 8:27–38).

Eunuchs were pitied by some. Sirach compared a person attempting to do right by violence to a eunuch lusting for sexual relations with a young woman—both were futile (Sir. 20:4). It is not clear if Sirach believed that eunuchs could not copulate. He also taught that one who was being punished by Yahweh and who was aware of what was happening could groan like a eunuch embracing a maiden (Sir. 30:20).

Jesus is reported to have stated that there were eunuchs who were born as eunuchs and were, presumably, without testicles, that there were those who were made eunuchs by castration, and that "there are those who have made themselves eunuchs for the sake of the kingdom of heaven" (Matt. 19:12). It is generally assumed that Jesus' statement should be taken metaphorically to refer to those who had become celibate or who had given up everything for the Christian faith. There is no evidence that Jesus' followers emulated the reported actions of males involved in some of the then-current mystery faiths, who in manic frenzy castrated themselves and offered their testicles to their deity.

Males are still concerned about protection of the genitals, and in sports special protective cups have been designed for such protection. There are occasions when one or more of the testicles must be removed because of disease or injury. Such individuals are not barred from the religious settings of their faith. However, lack of potency can be a factor in Roman Catholic marriages. For example, in January 1982, an Illinois man who was paralyzed and impotent was denied a Roman Catholic marriage because the man would not be able to consummate the marriage or, in the words of the priest, "fulfill his function as a husband." The couple wanted to be married in the parish church the woman had attended since childhood. Because there was no way to prove potency without engaging in premarital sexual activities, which are frowned on by the church, and because there were reported cases where paralyzed men had produced children, the hierarchy gave permission for the marriage.[1]

Vasectomy

Most attempts to control fertility in the Western world place the responsibility upon the woman. She is expected to be on the pill or to use a pessary, a diaphragm, or vaginal foam to prevent any sperm from making contact with the ovum. Males have used condoms since the time of Napoleon, but more recently some men have undergone a minor operation known as a vasectomy in which the sperm-carrying duct known as the vas deferens is severed just above the testes in the scrotum. The sperm is thus prevented from being ejaculated and is absorbed into the male body. For most men this operation has no side-effects, but some men are allergic to their own sperm and serious reactions affecting (in some cases) the thyroid have been experienced.

When some couples feel that they have produced all the children they wish to raise, the man, who may still be in his early thirties, may undergo a vasectomy. If the couple remain married, sexual relations become less complicated. The woman does not have to prepare for intercourse or to be on the pill; the man does not need to wear a condom. Intercourse is freer and more spontaneous. If the couple should divorce and the man remarries and wishes to have children by his new wife, the problem is complicated. An operation called a vaso-vasectomy is performed and the severed vas deferens are reconnected. If the time between the vasectomy and the vaso-vasectomy is not too great, the results are often satisfactory.

Some religious groups, including Jews, Roman Catholics, and some conservative Protestants, oppose the operation on the basis of the Deuteronomic legislation that prohibits a male whose testicles have been crushed to enter the sacred assembly (Deut. 23:1), or because humans are ''playing God'' and interfering with natural (God-given) processes. Of course the Roman Catholic church opposes all artificial means of preventing pregnancy and accepts only those methods that conform to the rhythms of the woman's fertility cycle. Just how sex during the infertile periods, which is obviously performed for pleasure and not for procreation, can be justified is difficult to understand. It is permissible to use natural (God-given) cycles to avoid fertilization but it is not permissible to use artificial (human-given) means. It is interesting that many Roman Catholics simply ignore the religious prohibitions.

NOTE

1. Reported in the *Los Angeles Times* by John Dart, religion writer, January 27, 1982.

11

Virginity

A virgin is a person who has never engaged in sexual intercourse. The person may have masturbated or have participated in heavy petting, but so long as there has been no actual intercourse that person is said to be a virgin. For the woman, the evidence of such abstinence has traditionally been an unbroken hymen. For the male, there is no physical evidence symbolizing chastity.

Virginity in the Bible

The writers of the Bible lay great emphasis upon the importance of virginity in women; no such emphasis is laid on virginity in males. Men are warned to stay away from an adulteress because they can get themselves into serious trouble (Prov. 7:6 ff.), but there is no demand that men be virgins when they marry.

So important was the unbroken hymen that the parents of the bride saved the bloodstained sheets from the daughter's wedding night as proof of her nuptial virginity. A case law preserved in Deuteronomy 22:13–21 states that if a man married a woman, "goes into her," and then became disaffected and charged her saying:

> I took this woman and when I approached her [sexually: drew into her] I found she was not a virgin [*bethulah*]

then the parents of the bride would produce "[the evidence of] the virginity of the young woman" (22:15), which consisted of her sleeping wrap or mantle (22:17). The cloth would be stained (one would hope) with blood from the ruptured hymen. If it were so stained, the man paid the girl's father 100 shekels for the shame he brought on the father and on the family for insinuating that the girl had not been protected from men. Furthermore, the man could never divorce the woman—she was his wife for life. If the sheets were not stained, the girl was killed outside of the city by stones hurled by the men of the city, because she had "played the whore" (22:21).

Virgin daughters were to be protected. There was fear that their lusting impulses could endanger their virginity. The sage Jesus, son of Sirach, wrote of his distrust of women:

A daughter brings her father secret insomnia
and worrying about her keeps him wakeful at night
if she is young that she fail to get married,
and if she is married, that she may become disliked.
When she is a virgin, lest she be violated
and become pregnant in her father's house
or when she has a husband that she may be unfaithful
or although married, lest she be barren.
Keep a close watch over a wayward daughter
lest she cause you to be a laughingstock for your enemies,
and make you a byword in the town and a mockery among the people,
causing you to be shamed before the public.
Do not permit her to parade her beauty before any man
nor take council with the women
for as out of clothes moths come
so out of women comes women's evil.
The evil of a man is better than the goodness of a woman,
for a woman brings confusion and shame.

[Sirach 42:9–14]

No such concern for virtue is expressed for a son, rather the emphasis is on instilling in the youth the proper respect for elders and behavior patterns that would lead to success in living.

For a woman, to be a virgin was to be unmarried, and to die unmarried and without having produced offspring was to die unfulfilled. This attitude is dramatically revealed in the story of Jephthah's daughter (Judg. 11). As the warrior leader of the Gileadite tribe of Hebrews, Jephthah vowed to Yahweh that, should he be victorious in battle against the Ammonites, he would sacrifice as a burnt offering "whoever comes out of the doors of my house to meet me when I return" (11:31). His only child, a daughter, came to meet him, rejoicing in his return with timbrels and dancing. However, Jephthah had made a vow. The daughter asked for a grace period of two months during which she would roam the hills with her companions and bewail her virginity. When she returned she was offered up as a burnt offering to Yahweh. As a commemoration, maidens in Israel each year spent four days bewailing the death of the young woman.

Folkloric parallels abound and the rite has been linked to fertility festivals.[1] The mourning ritual that included roaming the hills is a familiar motif that is mentioned in the myth of the god Ba'al found at ancient Ugarit. The goddess Anat, mourning the death of the fertility god Ba'al, wanders in the hills as she searches for the god's remains. Incidentally, she is called "the virgin Anat" (*bltlt 'nt*), but the term cannot mean that she did not have intercourse for the texts are quite explicit in describing her sexual relationship to the god Ba'al. Perhaps the term "virgin" was meant to imply her annual renewal as the goddess of fertility and the seasonal observation of her "marriage" to her brother Ba'al, the fertility god. She would be the perpetual virgin whose virginity was annually lost and then renewed.

The Hebrew word for virgin is *bethulah*, which may be derived from a Semitic root meaning "separation" or "apart," suggesting that the woman had been separated from or kept away from intimate association with males (Deut. 22:23; 2 Sam. 13:2). When the term *daughter* is added to *bethulah* ("virgin daughter") the phrase can be used to refer to the city of Jerusalem (Isa. 37:22; Jer. 14:17) or to foreign cities (Isa. 23:12, Sidon; 47:1, Babylon) perhaps implying that the cities had not been violated by invasion. One passage that at first glance seems to cloud the meaning of *bethulah* appears in Joel 1:8. A plague of locusts prompted a prophetic call for the people to lament as would a *bethulah* for her husband (*ba'al*), which may imply that the woman is now like a virgin without a man or, what is more likely, that the woman, a virgin, was betrothed. She could still refer to her husband-to-be as her *ba'al* and she would still be a *bethulah*, because no intercourse had occurred. The Greek equivalent term for *bethulah* is *parthenos*. In Christian scripture it is used to refer to both unmarried men and unmarried women (1 Cor. 7:25, 28, 34; Rev. 14:4).

The Hebrew word *almah* is derived from a Semitic root that appears to mean "to be sexually mature." The word does not indicate whether the person is or is not a virgin. It can be applied to both men and women. In 1 Samuel 20:22, Jonathan tells David how he will address his male servant, who is called a young man (*elem*). There is no way to tell whether the person was or was not a virgin. King Saul referred to David as an *elem* when he asked who the young man was who was confronting the Philistine strongman Goliath (1 Sam. 17:56). Abraham's servant told of his intention to stand by the well awaiting the *almah*, that is, the young woman who was sexually mature and who was presumably a virgin who would be Isaac's wife. The young women who played musical instruments in religious processions are called *almoth* in Psalm 68:26.

The Virgin Birth of Jesus

One of the more controversial passages in Jewish scripture involves the interpretation of the term *almah*. The prophet Isaiah was impatient with the vacillating posture of King Ahaz when the Judean monarch was confronted with imminent invasion from Israel and Syria. Isaiah demanded that Ahaz trust Yahweh and offered to provide a "sign" to demonstrate the divine promise of protection. Isaiah said:

Behold the *almah* will [is about to] conceive and bear a son and will call his name Immanuel. [Isaiah 7:14]

The statement does not make it clear whether or not the *almah* was a virgin at the moment of the prophetic utterance, but perhaps the implication that the birth was imminent suggests that she was not. The prophetic oracle continued with the assurance that before that child was old enough to know right from wrong the two enemies before whom Ahaz was trembling in fear would be eliminated. The promise is repeated in somewhat different form in Isaiah 8:1–4. In the Greek (Septuagint) translation of Isaiah 7:14, the term *parthenos* is used to translate *almah* rather than the Greek word *neanis*, which is a word that is closer in meaning and has almost the exact meaning of *almah*. Why the translators chose to translate *almah* with *parthenos* rather than *neanis* cannot be known now, but it is clear that for the translator in this particular passage *almah* meant *parthenos*. When the Christian writer of the Gospel of Matthew sought proof-texts from Jewish scripture to support his thesis that Jesus was the Messiah who fulfilled Jewish hopes, he used the Greek version of Isaiah 7:14 to support his belief that Jesus' birth was miraculous. He wrote:

Behold a *parthenos* will conceive and bear a son and his name will be called Emmanuel, which means God with us. [Matt. 1:23]

By using this passage from Isaiah, the gospel writer demonstrated his conviction that he had found prophetic substantiation for his belief that the Messiah, Jesus, was to be born of a virgin. The fact that the prophet Isaiah was addressing an eighth-century B.C.E. situation and was not concerned with the distant future is ignored by the gospel writer. He lifted the passage out of context and used it for his own purposes. Some Christian commentators have attempted to explain this gospel interpretation of the Isaiah passage by suggesting that the gospel writer, guided by the Holy Spirit, was provided with a new understanding and given a new meaning for the ancient prophecy. Of course, by the same argument, one could claim that the same Holy Spirit might give yet another new interpretation of the same passage today. But how does one test the Holy Spirit?

The virginity of Mary, the mother of Jesus, rests on other claims. In Matthew 1:18, the writer states that before the betrothed woman had experienced sexual intercourse with her husband, Joseph, she was found to be pregnant by the Holy Spirit. Should one wonder why Joseph would accept such a claim, Matthew explains that Joseph had a dream in which he was told that the male parent of the baby was the Holy Spirit (Matt. 1:20). Mary's virginity is also attested in the Gospel of Luke. She was told by the angel Gabriel that she was going to bear a child, and she asked, "How can this be, since I have not known a man [sexually]?" (Luke 1:34). She was told that her impregnation would be miraculous, that the Holy Spirit would "come upon" her, and that the power of the divine would "overshadow" her (Luke 1:35). Despite the sexual overtones that one might discover in this revelation, it is implied, perhaps, that the hymen would not be broken and that she would therefore technically still be a "virgin."

One might wonder why the early Christian community should have insisted upon the miraculous birth for Jesus and in particular a virgin birth. Hero figures in that time period were often accorded wondrous births. Isaac was born to Sarah when she was past ninety years of age (Gen. 18:21). Samson's mother was barren until an angel visited her and told her she would bear a child (Judg. 13), and the seer-prophet Samuel was born to Hannah after she had visited the shrine at Shiloh and prayed for a son (1 Sam. 1). Jesus' cousin, John the Baptizer, was born to an aged couple who had had no children and who, like Mary, were visited by the angel Gabriel (Luke 1). Sexual relationships between divine beings were common in hero stories. The Greek god Zeus impregnated women to produce heroes like Hercules, Perseus, and Alexander the Great. The god Apollo had intercourse with human females, who bore such heroes as Asclepius, Pythagoras, Plato, and the emperor Augustus. Some of the women were said to have been virgins. The use of mythological symbolism was part of the first-century literary tradition. The gospel writers simply used it to exalt Jesus. They could also find a reference in Jewish scripture to the impregnation of the human by the divine in the myth in Genesis 6:4, when the sons of God impregnated human females.

The Perpetual Virginity of Mary

The Roman Catholic church has made much of the "perpetual virginity" of Jesus' mother. References to Jesus' brothers, James, Joseph, Simon, and Judas, and to his sisters (Matt. 13:55–56), all of whom are accepted by non-Catholic scholars as children of Mary and Joseph, are explained as Joseph's children by a previous marriage, despite the fact that there is no gospel evidence for this claim. Some Catholics have pointed out that the term "brother" could be used to refer to an extended family to include cousins, thus the "brothers" might be cousins, sons of another Mary. The reference in Mark 3:20 to Jesus' "family" might symbolize his "family" of friends. The arguments are not convincing. There is no reason to believe that Joseph and Mary did not consummate their marriage and have sexual intercourse as did any other married Jewish couple who lived 2,000 years ago.

The purity of Mary was augmented in Roman Catholicism by the dogma of the Immaculate Conception, promulgated by Pope Pius XI in 1854. It was important to believe that Jesus was born of an immaculate, pure mother, one not even tainted by the "original sin" to which, according to Catholicism, all humans are heir. Mary, too, is miraculously born. For some Catholics the 1854 dogma acquired miraculous confirmation when in 1858 St. Bernadette (Soubirous), then a fourteen-year-old girl, had a vision of Mary, who told her: "I am the immaculate conception." The spring of water that welled up near or at the place of the revelation is now the site of the Lourdes shrine, where pilgrims go for healing in the "miraculously charged" waters. The combination of the emphasis on purity and the miraculous only enhances the traditional position of the Roman Catholic church on purity and chastity.

The emphasis on Mary's perpetual virginity betrays Christian uneasiness with the loss of the hymen—an uneasiness that originated in the Judaism out of which Christianity came. A good girl retained her hymen until she was penetrated by the penis of her husband. The Aaronic priests could marry only virgins, "They shall not take a whore-woman who has been pierced [deflorated] . . . " (Lev. 21:7) or a "widow or divorcee or one pierced or a whore," but only "a virgin [*bethulah*] from among his own people" (Lev. 21:14).

Virginity in the Early Church

For the early Christians, purity, chastity, and virginity were linked concepts. Paul wrote of the Christian church as the "virgin" bride (*parthenon hagnen*) of Christ, meaning an "undefiled" bride (2 Cor. 11:2). Men who had not been defiled by sexual associations with women were chaste (*parthenoi*) or virginal (Rev. 14:4). The early church put a premium on chastity and at the same time cast a shadow on sexual intercourse. Jesus was unmarried and was, presumably, a virgin despite continuing efforts in modern fiction to marry him off to suitable women, including Mary Magdalene.[2] Paul was not married and he too was, presumably, a virgin. He was convinced that he was living in the "last days" and that Jesus would soon return and establish the Kingdom of God (Christians only). He grudgingly (at least so it seems) gave his parishioners permission to marry, acknowledging that it was "better to marry than be on fire with passion" (1 Cor. 7:9). Those who were married (he counseled) should stay married and, although there was no sin in marriage, it was preferable to remain unmarried and devote oneself completely to preparation for the *parousia*—the Second Coming of Jesus (1 Cor. 7).

The Madonna-Whore

The sharp delineation between good and bad, chaste and unchaste, virginal and nonvirginal has provided the basis for what is commonly known as madonna-whore syndrome, which is often associated with sexual dysfunction. In the minds of some males, there are two kinds of women: the good and the bad, the chaste and the impure, the madonna and the whore. The whore is the one with whom one may enjoy sexual intimacies; the madonna is pure and on a pedestal above all lustful feelings, desires, and impulses. Such a man may be potent and have absolutely no sexual problems in clandestine affairs or in sex with a prostitute, but with his wife he may become impotent and be unable to get or maintain an erection. Women, too, can think in terms of the madonna-whore pattern, and those that do can become uncomfortable with their sexual feelings. For them, to experience desire is to be numbered with women who sell their bodies, with cheap women, with hussies who are sexually promiscuous. Sex is not quite clean or nice. She may feel so uncomfortable that she begins to create excuses to avoid sex with her husband. She may ultimately reach the point where participation in any sexual activity ceases.

Although sexual feelings are natural, attitudes toward sex are learned. Parents are role models for their children. The ways that the father relates to the mother and the mother to the father provide examples for the child of how men and women interact. In homes where there is virtually no talk about sex or where the talk is always in terms of the violation of mores, where the body is always hidden, where taboos about the body and its sexual functions are always present, the child learns restrictive and constrictive behavior. If such a home environment is augmented by strict religious training, young women can be trained to feel guilty about their sexual feelings and become convinced that orgasmic responses are sinful. Men become convinced that there are two kinds of women—those who are like their mothers, and perhaps also their sisters, who are pure, chaste, and undefiled, and are put on a pedestal, and those ''other'' women, who represent the sexual objects of male desire. Men marry women who represent the former and begin to experience impotency—how can one have sex with a madonna figure? They prove their virility with the latter.

Sex therapy often involves a re-learning experience involving the discovery by the male that his chaste partner is really a ''total'' woman with normal passions, desires, and responses. For the wife who has madonna images of herself, it is important to learn that it is permissible to enjoy her body and be free and enthusiastic in her sexual relations with her husband. She learns that it is normal to experience the physical and emotional ecstasy of orgasm.

The degree to which religious beliefs help to develop the madonna-whore imagery cannot be reckoned. Within Catholicism the emphasis on the purity of Mary as an ideal for womanhood has significant impact:

> For the young boy, Mary is the symbol of the wise, perfect woman, and in the confused emotional feelings of adolescence he instinctively turns to her gracious serenity for consolation and strength. She is at once a saint of dazzling virtue and a loving mother, and the example of her pure chastity has helped many a boy and girl.
>
> A little later the young man's attitude becomes more that of a chivalrous knight—an attitude which is reflected in his dealings with all other women. The fact that womanhood is accorded such an honorable place in Christian teaching is mainly due to the devotion to Our Lady.[3]

Within Judaism and Christianity there is a continuing emphasis on chastity and virginity. There are many young people who enter into marriage relationships as virgins but are not uninformed about sexual behavior. Having been introduced to varying aspects of human sexuality through courses in health education, they have supplemented their course work by extensive reading and often by consultation with marriage counselors. They enter into their marriage as virgins, but as informed virgins.

The Unbroken Hymen at the End of the Twentieth Century

The unbroken hymen can no longer be accepted as the proof of virginity in women. Hymens can be stretched and torn in a number of ways that have nothing to do with sexual intercourse, including the insertion of tampons. Some hymens are thick, some are thin, some practically cover the vaginal opening, some are almost nonexistent. Still, in some parts of the world, the hymen remains as the token of female virginity. Among some Christian Copts in Egypt, the bride is examined by a matron who inserts a finger into the vagina to see if blood can be drawn. Among the Muslims of upper Egypt, the nuptial sheets are expected to show the bloody evidence of the torn hymen. But women who have had premarital sex have found ways to deceive the "hymen-happy." In Iran, the torn membrane can be temporarily stitched with needle and thread. Wise women in upper Egypt provide tiny capsules of chicken blood to be used by the bride on her wedding night. Of course there are equally wise women who have stated that they can distinguish between human and chicken blood!

Punishment of the bride whose hymen has been broken before marriage has almost been outmoded, but there are places where it still persists. The woman may be disinherited by her family and rejected by the bridegroom. She may be cast out to make her own way in a society that is hostile to premarital sex and that therefore almost compels her to become a prostitute to survive. There are some few who would kill her for bringing shame on herself and the family.

Among modern teen-agers, the unbroken hymen can be something of a curiosity. There is often peer pressure to lose virginity on both men and women. Those who haven't "made it" yet are sometimes made to feel that they are out of step with the times. The emphasis among some teen-aged men on "scoring" often gives rise to fabrications about sexual exploits. Among young women, the question "Are you still a virgin?" can carry the unspoken query "Whatever is wrong with you?"

Young women of college age often bow to peer pressure and decide it is time to lose their virginity. They deliberately seek a male to assist them. It is not surprising that on their initial encounter many find sex greatly overrated. Their male partners are often inexperienced, overeager, clumsy, insensitive, and sometimes downright crude. The sorority girl who decided it was time to experience sexual intercourse finally "gave in" to a young man from a neighboring fraternity whom she had dated for several weeks and who was pressuring her to "make love." He returned to his fraternity house after midnight, where his loud triumphant cries roused any sleeping "brothers" as he boasted, "I got me a real live virgin, an untouched one, but she ain't a virgin no more!" He went to sleep that night with the complements of his fraternity brothers ringing in his ears. The next day the girl, who was still unsure about what she had experienced, learned of his chauvinistic boast. What had been a significant decision for her was turned into a cheap moment of having been involved in nothing more than "making out."

But not all young men and women yield to peer pressure and popular trends; a significant number remain virgins until the time of marriage. A recent study has shown that regular church attendance and involvement in religious activities and conformity to conservative parental norms are demonstrable factors in maintaining virginity in women between the ages of sixteen and twenty-two.[4] Within religious settings, peer-group pressure may be to conform to the acceptance of maintaining virginity, thereby reducing the impact of other influences encouraging sexual involvement outside of marriage.

Some men who engage in sexual intercourse before marriage still plan to marry virgins. The old double-standard in sex mores persists. Perhaps there is some insecurity in the male who feels constantly called upon to perform. He wonders what his partner's former bedfellows may have been like as lovers. His need for reassurance that the past is the past and that only the present matters, or that he is truly the best lover, can put toxic demands upon the woman and become pathological in the man. For such insecure males, perhaps it is best to marry a virgin; there are no past lovers to compete with.

Virginity is still important in Western culture. Many young people are "saving it" for the marriage bed. They are not ignorant about sex. They know what it is about and what they are expected to do in making love, but they are willing to wait to share the experience with someone who is of the utmost importance to them and who will be a lifetime partner, not just a one-night stand.

On the other hand, many modern weddings are between couples who are not virgins. Both partners have had previous sexual experience—sometimes with other persons and sometimes between themselves in premarital intercourse. They accept one another in love and do not worry about what has been. What matters most are the feelings that exist between them now.

There are no relevant statistics to demonstrate that marriages between virgins is a better or more lasting arrangement than marriage between nonvirgins. Our culture is open to both.

NOTES

1. Theodor H. Gaster, *Myth, Legend and Custom in the Old Testament* (New York, 1969, 1975), vol. 2 pp. 430–32.

2. See, for example, M. Baigent, R. Leigh, and H. Lincoln, *Holy Blood, Holy Grail*. (New York, 1982).

3. N. G. M. Van Doornik, S. Jelsma, A. Van de Lisdonk (ed. by John Greenwood), *The Handbook of the Catholic Faith* (New York, 1954, 1956–1962), p. 243.

4. Edward S. Herold and Marilyn S. Goodwin, "Adamant Virgins, Potential Nonvirgins and Nonvirgins," *Journal of Sex Research* May 1981, pp. 97–113.

12

Celibacy

Celibacy is the state of being unmarried. It implies that the individual does not engage in sexual activity. The prophet Jeremiah lived a celibate life. He did so because he believed that this life-style was in accord with the will of Yahweh:

> The word of Yahweh came to me: You shall not take a wife nor shall you have sons and daughters in this place [Jer. 16:1]

Whether or not the phrase "in this place" was meant to suggest that Jeremiah married and had children in some other place, perhaps in Egypt, where he was taken by the Jews after the destruction of Jerusalem, cannot be known (Jer. 43:6).

There were others who became celibates for religious reasons. The Essenes, according to Philo (*Hypothetica* 11:14), abstained from sexual relations. More information has come from the Dead Sea Scrolls, the literature found near what is believed to have been the Essene headquarters, located at Qumran at the northwest corner of the Dead Sea. This sect of Jews believed they were involved in a new covenant with Yahweh. They believed that they, as the Children of Light, would be involved in the final eschatological battle with Belial and the Children of Darkness. Their community was conceived of as an army encampment and subject to the regulations governing sexual involvement during war as set forth in the Torah (Deut. 23:9–14). After engaging in sexual relations a Jew was considered to be unclean until evening (Lev. 15:18) and would of necessity be barred from the encampment, which consisted of volunteers committed to keeping the camp undefiled in preparation for the holy war. To prevent possible defilement or impurity that might come from sexual association with a woman and which would cause the withdrawal of divine support, the Children of Light eschewed marriage.

John the Baptizer was unmarried. Apparently he too felt a commitment to the celibate life because of his sense of a divine calling. Jesus and some of his followers, including the apostle Paul, were celibate. When Jesus was asked by his disciples whether it was better for a man to remain single if divorce was forbidden and there was no escape from an unhappy marriage, Jesus responded that "not every man can accept this saying, but only those to whom it is given.'' He then pointed out that some were born eunuchs, some were castrated, some became eunuchs ''for the sake of the kingdom of heaven,'' and he concluded with ''he who is able to accept this, let him accept it'' (Matt. 19:1–12). In other words, Jesus did not demand celibacy from his followers; it was only for those who could accept it (assuming of course that he was not suggesting castration!). Jesus praised those who would forsake family, including wife and children, for the sake of the kingdom of God (Luke 18:29), which meant the acceptance of the celibate way of life for a religious cause (see also Luke 14:26). Paul, who was celibate, wished his followers could be as he was (1 Cor. 7:7).

The precepts of Jesus and the Essene community fly in the face of traditional Jewish thought, which placed a premium on marriage and the family. Nevertheless, Jeremiah was not condemned when he practiced celibacy. Individuals and perhaps especially ascetics were accepted for their beliefs.

It is not surprising to find within Western Christianity a strong emphasis on celibacy of the clergy. The biblical basis for this custom is Matthew 19:11. Voluntary continence permits the clergy to concentrate on religious matters and the work of the kingdom of God without being burdened by family responsibilities. Although celibacy is demanded of priests in Roman Catholicism (with some exceptions), the Eastern churches permit marriage for deacons and priests but bar married persons from becoming bishops.

How do celibates deal with their natural sexual impulses? Generally these libidinous feelings are suppressed or sublimated and redirected into other interests and activities. This was not always the pattern among Roman Catholic clergy. At certain periods priests were permitted conjugal relationships, although celibacy was the ideal. In other times, ''spiritual marriages'' were allowed and the priest and his ''spiritual mate'' would live together and perhaps share the same bed while remaining chaste. The history of the church is pock-marked with transgressions of the celibate rule by male and female clergy and even today one learns of individuals who violate their vows.

Most celibate clergy learn to control their desires. They become very busy with their duties and responsibilities and bury themselves in work, which leaves little time for lustful thoughts. They pray and through worship and devotion to their calling attempt to control their thoughts and feelings. Most are successful. The longer they persist in the celibate way of life, the weaker the libidinous demands become. The axiom ''use it or lose it'' functions well for them.

Some married couples practice temporary celibacy in accordance with the teachings of Paul, the apostle, who recommended abstinence for a time devoted to prayer (1 Cor. 7:5). Some couples believe that temporary continence enhances one's sex life.

13

Menstruation

Menstrual taboos can be found in almost every culture. Whether they are to be explained as originating from male blood phobia (Freud) or as being linked with some external magical power tied to the phases of the moon, with other natural phenomena, or with the natural forces associated with fertility, or whether they represent primitive man's confusion over the fact that despite loss of blood the woman did not weaken and die, or by any one or more of the numerous proposed explanations, it really does not matter; the taboo exists.

There are a number of references to menstruation in the Bible and all are negative. Because the Bible was written by males, the passages reflect male discomfort with menstruation and menstrual blood—a discomfort that goes so far as to render the menstruating woman ceremonially unclean, sexually off limits and unacceptable, and socially isolated.

The Menstrual Rag

The menstrual rag is a symbol of that which is unclean and is to be cast away. In an addition made centuries later to the writings of the eighth-century B.C.E. prophet Isaiah of Jerusalem, an author portrayed a new purified Jerusalem. He wrote:

> Then you will defile your silver-plated carved images and your gold-plated molded images. You will cast them away like a menstrual rag saying to them: Go away! [Isa. 30:22]

The command "go away" or "disappear" or "be gone" may reflect a magical formula associated with the disposal of the bloodied menstrual rags pronounced by a woman at the close of her period. She cleanses herself of that which renders her unclean.

The Greek version of the Book of Esther includes material that does not appear in the Hebrew text. These extra verses are part of the Roman Catholic Version and can be found in the Apocrypha of Protestantism and Judaism. In Roman Catholicism, they hold the same authoritative position as the rest of the Bible. In a prayer, Esther tells her god of her distaste for the role she feels she must play: a Jewish woman who is a queen in a pagan Persian court. She says:

> You know I am under pressure, that I abhor the symbol of high rank that I wear upon my head when I appear in public—I abhor it like a menstrual rag and do not wear it in private. [Esther 14:16]

Menstrual rags were private garments and not for public display, even as pads and tampons are today. To describe the crown of Persia as the equivalent of a menstrual rag being worn on the head underscores both the discomfort Esther felt in wearing it and the feeling of revulsion associated with the menstrual rag.

Contamination

In the laws of the Torah that deal with bodily emissions, a woman is declared "unclean" during her seven-day menstrual period. Everything and everyone she comes in contact with is defiled (Lev. 15:19–24). Moreover, anyone who touches anything she has contaminated also becomes impure and must undergo rituals of cleansing. If a man copulates with her, he contracts her impurity and becomes unclean for a period of seven days. Indeed, the Levitical legislation demands excommunication of both partners for sexual relations during menstruation (Lev. 20:18).

Should the flow of blood continue beyond the prescribed seven days, or be continuous, the woman is unclean so long as the blood flows and she retains her contaminatory potential (Lev. 15:25–27). After the flow of blood has ceased, the woman must wait for seven days and make two offerings—one for sin and the other as a whole burnt-offering. The correlation between sin and ritual uncleanness is clear. Indeed, one of the sins listed by Ezekiel as contributing to divine judgment and the destruction of Jerusalem was sexual relations during menstruation (Ezek. 22:10).

Because of her contaminatory potential, a woman was isolated during menstruation. Only after ritual cleansing was she purified and available for sexual intercourse. It was when Bathsheba, the wife of Uriah the Hittite, one of King David's soldiers, was washing herself at the end of her menstrual period that David copulated with her (2 Sam. 11:2–4).

One can only imagine the plight of the woman with a continuing flow of blood. A woman who had had a problem of blood-flow for twelve years is said to have been magically healed simply by touching the hem of Jesus' robe (Matt. 9:20–22 and parallels). No reference is made to cleansing rites, nor does Jesus appear to have been polluted by the contact. The story is one in a sequence of accounts demonstrating the power of faith.

In one of the patriarchal legends associated with Jacob, the menstrual taboo plays an important role. Jacob became aware that his father-in-law, Laban, had changed his attitude toward him and that his brothers-in-law were disaffected because they feared that Jacob would inherit Laban's property. Jacob took his wives Leah and Rachel and fled. Before leaving, Rachel stole her father's *teraphim*. The *teraphim* were small idols that may have been used in divination but also were vitally important in the transference of property. Indeed, the inheritor of the land had to have the figurines in hand to establish a claim. By stealing these idols, Rachel was securing property rights for her husband.

Laban overtook them and began to search their tents for his idols. When he entered Rachel's tent he found her sitting on a camel saddle under which she had hidden the *teraphim*. She asked to be left as she was because "the way of women is upon me," that is, "I am in my period." Laban respected the taboo associated with this condition and left her as she was, without becoming contaminated by touching her. He did not find the stolen idols. The legend contains no mention of the requirements for ritual cleansing that were part of Hebrew-Jewish cultic law.

The taboo has not faded within Western culture despite modern knowledge about this female cyclic pattern. Ancient laws can still be evoked; ancient beliefs can still affect the sexual behavior of moderns. For example, within Orthodox Judaism, a woman must still refrain from sex until seven days have passed after the termination of her period and until she has taken a ritual bath (*mikveh*). The ritual bath may be taken in any water deep enough to immerse the entire body from head to toe. Specially prepared basins or baths called *mikvas* are deep enough so that the water reaches the breasts and they are found in almost every Orthodox Jewish community. Every hair of the woman's head must go beneath the water. Prior to the washing, the man keeps as great a distance from the woman as possible for fear of contamination.

In our culture, where it is customary to shake hands when being introduced, one socially active Orthodox rabbi always excuses himself to women with a diverting sexist comment: "I never start anything I don't finish, so I will not touch you." If he were as honest as he is courtly he would admit that he is afraid that the woman might be in her menstrual period and he would inadvertently be contaminated.

The power of the taboo against sex during menstruation is apparent in a case reported by Masters and Johnson. An Orthodox Jew was unable to ejaculate intravaginally because at the age of 24 he had attempted to force physical attention upon a young woman who stopped him by saying she was menstruating. Although he never saw her again, the trauma associated with the near-violation of taboo affected him so severely that a marriage of eight years was not consummated.[1]

These same authors describe the case of a woman raised in a fundamentalist Protestant home where absolutely no information about sex was given or was available. She was absolutely unprepared for the onset of menstruation, which was explained by her mother in terms of "the curse." One can only imagine the bewilderment of a child who is instructed that menstruation was something she had to endure, and told that there would be pain.[2]

In 1970, the Roman Catholic church in America invoked the ancient laws of Leviticus to prevent women from serving in the sanctuary as lectors or commentators during the Mass. This is not a new concern, but is part of the history of barring women from leadership within the church.[3] Folklore is also still current within certain groups and families about menstruous women turning milk sour, causing weakness in men who copulate with them, affecting the luck at a gambling table or in some financial venture, making creative persons uncreative, and so on. Of course there is absolutely no scientific evidence for these beliefs.

The biblical restrictions on sex during menstruation reflect the attitude of a group of people who lived several thousand years ago and who recorded their cultural and religious attitudes and biases toward menstruation. Modern studies have shown that there is absolutely no physical reason for not engaging in sexual relations during a woman's menstrual period, unless the woman experiences some discomfort. Indeed, some women, and some men, experience heightened pleasure at this particular time. It has been suggested that aesthetic reasons might make some hesitant to engage in sexual encounters during a woman's menstrual period. Aesthetic responses are learned and are culturally induced. They can be by-passed and unlearned if a couple so desires.

Pre-menstrual Stress

Until recently, most medical studies about the menstrual period were published by men, who of course do not menstruate. In some studies mention was made of pre-menstrual tensions, and it was recorded that some women complained of physical pain, including migraine headaches, cramps, backaches, and so on, and some talked of emotional difficulties, such as shortness of temper and feelings of anger. There was a tendency to suggest that the complaints were more imaginary than real. New studies, particularly those made by women, explain these changes in feelings of well-being, both physical and mental, in terms of chemical changes within the woman's body that have both physical and emotional affects. These varying complaints and symptoms have now been grouped under what is known as the pre-menstrual syndrome, or, more familiarly, PMS. It is now known that the menstrual cycle is activated by the pituitary gland and that profound changes take place within the woman's body in a remarkable biological process—a process that has been described over and over again in books about human sexuality and menstruation. The process is normal and natural. There is nothing unnatural or supernatural about it. It is part of the normal cycle of a woman's life. Some women have more physically painful reactions than others; some have deeper emotional responses. Each person is an individual and the PMS will vary from person to person. Women and, it is hoped, men learn to cope with the changes.

The "Curse"

Menstruation is sometimes referred to as the "curse," as though there were something supernatural about it. Sometimes the "curse" is related to the punishment imposed upon Eve in the Genesis creation myth (Gen. 2:4–3, 24). According to this myth, Adam and Eve were in an idyllic setting in the Garden of Eden. They were to act as caretakers for the divine estates of the Hebrew god Yahweh. They were permitted to eat of any tree in the garden, with the exception of the "tree of knowledge of good and evil." Eve, tempted by a serpent, ate of the forbidden tree, gave some of the fruit to Adam, and both were expelled from the garden before they could eat of the tree of immortality and live forever. In actuality, Eve and Adam were not cursed; they were punished. Eve's punishment was:

> I will make your child-bearing pain intense; in pain you will bear children. Yet your [sexual] urge will be for your husband and he will continue to cause you to bear [master you]. [Gen. 3:16]

The punishment was pain in childbirth and subservience to the male—a severe punishment indeed, but one that had nothing to do with menstruation. This creation myth, written by male Hebrews, indicates that women's secondary role came about by divine ordinance and was punishment for Eve's disobedience.

NOTES

1. William H. Masters and Virginia E. Johnson, *Human Sexual Inadequacy* (Boston, 1970), pp. 117 f.

2. Ibid. pp. 230 f.

3. Sr. Albertus Magnus McGrath, O.P., *What a Modern Catholic Believes About Women* (Chicago, 1972), p. 22; Clara Maria Henning, "Canon Law and the Battle of the Sexes," in *Religion and Sexism*, ed. by Rosemary Reuther (New York, 1974), pp. 272 ff.

14

Adultery

Adultery is voluntary sexual intercourse between a married person and someone other than his or her spouse. Because marriage presumes an exclusive relationship between partners, adultery is a betrayal of that bond. It is condemned in the Bible and forbidden by Jews, Christians, and Muslims, although within each of these groups there are those who engage in adulterous relationships.

Adultery in Jewish Scriptures

The seventh commandment of the Decalogue is abrupt and to the point: "You shall not commit adultery" (Exod. 20:14; Deut. 5:18) and the law applies to both men and women. Violation was punishable by death if the couples were caught in the act. Leviticus 20:10 reads, "If a man commits adultery with his neighbor's wife, both the adulterer and the adulteress shall be killed." The law appears also in Deuteronomy 22:23 f. but in a somewhat expanded form. If a betrothed virgin (who was the equivalent of a married woman) copulates with a man in a city or a town, both parties are killed. The point at issue is that the woman could not claim she was raped, for in the town she could cry out for help. If the intercourse took place in the fields, away from the settled area, it was assumed that the woman was raped and only the man was killed.

The emphasis in the laws and in the narratives that refer to rape or potential rape is often upon the woman as property of the male. Adultery is, therefore, violation of property belonging to another. Not only is a criminal act involved but also a moral offense that brought shame to the husband or to the woman's family for failing to manage to protect the woman.

One Abrahamic legend tells of Abraham's representing Sarah as his sister rather than as his wife, resulting in Sarah being in bed with King Abimelech. Before sexual intercourse could take place, the monarch learned by divine revelation that Sarah was married. He reacted in horror and accused Abraham of nearly bringing a "great sin" on him and the kingdom (Gen. 20:9). So serious was the violation of the marriage vow that when a king was involved the deity could punish the nation, even though the king as the adulterer was completely innocent and believed that the woman was single.

The saga of Joseph tells of the patriarch as a young man in Egypt, where he was a slave in the house of one of Pharaoh's eunuchs named Potiphar (Gen. 39). Potiphar's wife became enamoured of the young man and invited him to "come and have intercourse with me" ("lie with me"). Joseph resisted and appealed to her sense of honor, pointing out the trust Potiphar had in Joseph. He asked, "How can I do such a wicked thing and sin against God?" She continued to pressure him and one day grabbed Joseph's cloak and again invited him to "come and have intercourse with me." The young man fled, leaving his cloak behind. The frustrated woman accused him of rape. (See Chapter 16.) In both patriarchal narratives, there is emphasis upon the seriousness of adultery as the violation of a divine command.

When a man was suspicious of his wife and believed she was sexually involved with another, it was up to him to take action (Num. 5:11–28). He was to bring her before the priest, together with the appropriate barley-meal offering. What follows is an incredible mixture of superstition and magic. The priest unbound or let down the woman's hair—a ritual that is not really understood but that seems to have been associated with mourning rites. He took "holy water" (which could mean water that had been blessed, water from some holy spring, or water from a sanctuary container) in a clay pot and mixed into it dust from the sanctuary floor. The barley meal, which is called "the memory offering" and "the jealousy offering," was placed in the woman's hands. The priest carried the water and dust mixture, which was called "the bitter waters that bring the curse." After making the woman take an oath, which is not given in the biblical text, the priest recited a magical incantation:

> If no man has copulated ["lain"] with you, and if you have not defiled yourself [by adultery] while under your husband's authority, be free from this bitter water that brings the curse. But if you have gone astray while under your husband's authority, and if you are defiled and some man other than your husband has copulated with you . . . Yahweh make you a curse and an execration among your people when Yahweh makes your thigh fall away [miscarriage?] and your body swell [pregnancy?] may this water that brings the curse pass through your bowels and make your body swell [pregnancy?] and your thigh fall away [miscarriage?]. And the woman shall say amen, amen [so let it be].

Next the priest wrote the curses on a tablet and washed them off into the bitter water and made the woman drink it. He took the barley meal from her hand and waved it before the altar, burned some of it, then brought the waters to the woman again and made her drink. If the woman was guilty of adultery, the "bitter waters," now magically empowered both by the dust from the sanctuary floor and by the ink that carried the curse, would cause pain, an unwanted pregnancy, and miscarriage. If she was not guilty, then she would conceive children normally by her husband.

Throughout the trial, the woman is presumed guilty until proven innocent. The use of incantations, magically empowered water, and ritual, all designed to terrify the woman, has sadistic overtones. The text states clearly that the woman was under her husband's control. She has no choice but to obey and go through the rite. There was no condemnation of the husband if the woman was found innocent and no attempt to involve her sex partner if she was judged guilty. Primitive magical notions are apparent in these particular biblical texts. The dirt from the sanctuary floor, believed to have some potency because it was from a place considered to be holy, was nothing more than plain dust. Holy water, whether from a sacred spring or from someplace in the tabernacle, or even if blessed by the priest, remained nothing more than plain water. The magical incantation that was to cause the deity to affect the woman's body could only affect the woman if she believed in its efficacy. Studies in primitive witchcraft and demonology have demonstrated the effectiveness of such mumbo-jumbo among people who believed in magic and in the supernatural powers of the priesthood or the witchdoctors. Apparently such rites were part of the Hebrew culture during the fifth century B.C.E., when this particular writing is believed to have been recorded.

The wise man who instructed his male students in the words of Proverbs 6:32–35 provided another point of view:

> He who commits adultery with a woman has no sense
> And he who presses her is self destructive.
> He will get wounds and dishonor
> And his disgrace will not be wiped away.
> For jealousy enrages a husband
> And he will show no mercy when he takes revenge
> Nor will he accept compensation
> Or be appeased if you give him many gifts.

Here the focus is on the man and what might happen to him if he is caught. He will not only face the fury of a cuckolded husband, but his reputation will suffer too. The words of the wise men were almost always on practical results, not on theological significance, but there were exceptions. Sirach, whose school flourished during the second century B.C.E., warned his students against the attitude of those who thought they were getting away with adultery:

> A man who commits adultery in his own bed and says in his heart [thinks] "Who sees me? The walls of my house conceal me, the roof overshadows me, so no one sees me. So what is to hinder me from sinning?" [Sirach 23:18]

Sirach warns that the deity, whose eyes are "ten thousand times brighter than the sun," perceives the hidden ways of mortals. Punishment will come in the open street when the man is least ready for it.

According to one writer in Proverbs, the adulteress may also dismiss her behavior as insignificant:

> This is the way of an adulterous woman:
> she eats, wipes her mouth
> and says, "I have done no wrong."

[Prov. 30:20]

Apparently not everyone felt guilt for violating a law believed to have been given by the deity, or an ethic approved by the society.

Sirach also condemns the woman who leaves her husband and produces a child by a stranger. He notes that she has disobeyed a divine law, committed an offense against her husband, committed adultery, and produced an illegitimate child. Sirach believed that her children would never mature and have families and her memory would be a curse, while she herself would be brought before the assembly for judgment (Sirach 23:22–27).

Another Jew, who is believed to have lived in Alexandria, Egypt, during the first century B.C.E., wrote in the name of King Solomon, the wise king. His wisdom sayings are included in the Roman Catholic and Eastern Orthodox Bibles under the title "Wisdom" (of Solomon) but are not accepted as authoritative by Jews and Protestants. He taught that:

> Children of adulterers will remain without offspring
> and products of an unlawful intercourse will die.
> Even if they should live a long life, they will be held in low esteem
> and, in the end, their old age will be without honor.
> If they die young, they will have no hope
> nor comfort in the time of judgment.

[Wisdom 3:16–18]

This writer adds two new dimensions to the condemnation of adultery: the curse that falls on the children born from the adulterous relationship and the threat that the children will have no comfort when the final day of judgment comes. The idea of afterlife and judgment in the afterlife came into Judaism during the late Persian and early Greek periods (fourth to second centuries B.C.E.). Divine judgment falls on the children who had no part in the adulterous affair.

For the prophets, the yielding of the Hebrews to the lure of the fertility cults was not only apostasy but adultery, for Israel was the "wife" of Yahweh in the imagery of Hosea, Jeremiah,and Ezekiel (Hos. 2:2 f., 13, 14; Jer. 23:14; 29:23). The prophets could refer back to the commandments as divinely given guides to conduct (Jer. 7:9–10), but the people went their own way. It was the conviction of the prophets that disobedience to the revealed law could only bring punishment from Yahweh in the form of national disaster. Certainly Ezekiel interpreted the destruction of Jerusalem and the Babylonian captivity in that light.

But punishment, both social and divine was not always inflicted, at least not always in an obvious way, on the perpetrators. *Post-eventum* insight could provide a convenient explanation. David's relationship with Bathsheba began as an adulterous affair (2 Sam. 11). The king observed Bathsheba bathing, invited (ordered?) her to come to the palace, had intercourse with her, and when he found she was pregnant attempted to have her husband have intercourse with her so that David would not be recognized as the father of the child. Uriah, Bathsheba's husband, was a loyal Hebrew soldier. He accepted the naive Hebrew superstition that association with a woman would somehow negatively affect the war, so he slept in the barracks rather than spending the time with his wife. David had him killed in battle so that he and Bathsheba could marry. The child born of the adulterous relationship was weak and ill. David went through the pretense of grieving in the hope that he might influence Yahweh to spare the child's life. When the child died, David immediately returned to his normal patterns of life. The prophet Nathan interpreted the death of the child as divine judgment and punishment for David's behavior, which could be judged as murderous or adulterous, or both. The next child born to David and Bathsheba was Solomon, who succeeded David to the throne.

The story of Susanna and the elders is about a false accusation of adultery. This tale is included in the Roman Catholic Bibles as part of the book of Daniel but is rejected by Jews and Protestants as a noncanonical document. Susanna was the wife of a prominent Jew named Joakim who regularly opened his home to the Jewish community. Two Jewish elders lusted after her and schemed to have sexual relations with her. They accused her of adultery with an unidentified young man whom they said they had witnessed with her in Joakim's garden. She was judged, and condemned to death. As she was being led to her execution, Daniel, who at that time was a very young man, came to her rescue. He questioned the elders separately, found discrepancies in their stories, and exonerated Susanna.

Death was the accepted penalty for adultery. King David escaped civil judgment. The divine punishment that should have fallen upon him allegedly fell upon the child born of the adulterous union, and that child died. Nor was Bathsheba punished for her part in the adulterous relationship, perhaps because of David's status. Susanna would have been killed, despite the fact that she was innocent, on the basis of the trumped-up story of two lecherous witnesses had she not been rescued by Daniel.

Adultery in Christian Scriptures

The Christian scriptures record a legend in which Jesus encountered a group of Jews of the Pharisee sect who were about to stone a woman caught in the act of adultery (John 7:53–8:11). Jesus rescued her from death by suggesting that only a Jew who was guiltless should cast the first stone. No stones were thrown. Jesus did not condemn the woman.

The story is romantic and beautiful but is most likely a legend without any historical foundation. It does not appear in any manuscripts of the Gospel of John before the fifth century C.E. It is probably a trumped-up story reflecting what some Christians felt Jesus would have said in such a situation. Despite its strong emphasis on forgiveness, it has not been of major importance in the Christian approach to the issue of adultery.

Adultery is condemned in Christian scriptures just as it was in Jewish writings. When a young man approached Jesus and asked him what he must do to inherit eternal life, Jesus referred to the commandments, including the prohibition against adultery (Mark 10:19 and parallels). The apostle Paul also refers to the Decalogue in listing the essentials of a moral life (Rom. 13:9). The Jewish attitude toward adultery was also the Christian attitude—it was against the will of the deity. Those who commit adultery will be judged by the deity (Heb. 13:4) and will be excluded from the kingdom of heaven (1 Cor. 6:9).

But within the Christian scriptures, adultery is given a new definition. A divorced person who remarries while the first spouse is still living commits adultery. The Gospel of Mark reports Jesus' response to the Pharisees who asked him if it was lawful for a man to divorce his wife. Jesus asked them what the Mosaic law required. When they told him that a man could write up a certificate of divorce for his wife, Jesus said that it was because of the hard-heartedness of the people that Moses had given the prescription. He argued that what "God has joined together, let no man separate." His disciples questioned him further about his teaching and he said:

> Whoever divorces his wife and marries another commits adultery against her. And if she divorces her husband and marries another she commits adultery. [Mark 10:10–12].

Both Matthew and Luke, who used Mark's work in their writing, omit the reference to the wife divorcing the husband. Indeed, Luke omits the whole conversation and only gives Jesus' teaching:

> Every man who divorces his wife and marries another commits adultery, and he who marries a woman divorced from her husband commits adultery. [Luke 16:18].

The Markan account is abbreviated in Matthew 19:3–9, and the regulation is softened by the addition of the words "except for fornication":

> . . . every man who divorces his wife, except on the grounds of fornication [unchastity] makes her an adulteress, and whoever marries a divorced woman commits adultery. [Matt. 5:32; cf. Matt. 19:9].

It was not long ago that there was some attempt to enforce the Matthean regulation on divorce in the Western world. People who had married, only to discover they were incompatible and were miserable together, were not permitted a divorce except on the ground of unchastity. In Canada it was not uncommon for the couple to agree on a procedure: the man would go to a cheap hotel and hire a woman (often an actress) to pose in her bra with him. He would have his shirt off, but pants on. A photographer and a private detective would open the door, take a picture, and everyone would go home. The picture would be used in court as evidence of the husband's sexual dalliance with another woman. The Canadian government had to face a reality: whether it was wiser to let couples divorce for reasons other than adultery or to continue to force people who were unhappy together to choose between remaining married or becoming liars in court. They relaxed the divorce laws. With the adultery charge gone, it was no longer important for gossips to know who preferred the charges so that the "guilty party" might be properly identified.

Not every Christian group pays much attention to the New Testament teachings on divorce. Marriage within the Greek Orthodox church is a sacrament and is entered into for life. The marriage can be dissolved by the church on the basis of fornication, and civil divorces with the privilege of remarriage are recognized.[1] Roman Catholic marriage is also a sacrament, and because the church believes that God dissolved the marriage between Hagar and Abraham and gave Moses a law for dissolution (Deut. 24:1) the pope has the power to dissolve marriages, but only where the marriage has never been consummated. All other marriages if they are "sacramentally consecrated and consummated can never be dissolved."[2] Civil divorces of such consecrated marriages are not recognized by the church. Within Mormonism, marriage is a solemn agreement that extends beyond the grave into eternity; but, although divorce is discouraged, temple divorces are granted.

Both Jewish and Christian groups discourage divorce, but most are willing to accept it when it occurs. Nor is there any public labeling in Christian churches of those who have divorced and remarried. When the Worldwide Church of God, in Pasadena, attempted to enforce the gospel teachings about remarriage after divorce as the equivalent of adultery, the opposition from the parishioners caused the church leaders to back down. Fundamentalists and evangelical Christians of the far Right carefully avoid references to these passages, because to emphasize them would indict and estrange a large percentage of their supporters and decimate their congregations.

This same group carefully avoids the label "adultery" when referring to the divorce and remarriage of prominent people they hope to influence. For example, when the Reverend Tim LaHaye, co-founder of the so-called Moral Majority, was asked in a public forum in San Diego whether, on the basis of his belief in the authority of the New Testament as the divinely revealed "Word of God," if he believed that President Reagan, who is divorced and remarried, was an adulterer, LaHaye weaseled out of the question and said, "I think God will forgive President Reagan." For what the President of the United States would be forgiven was not clear. Was it for being an adulterer under Jesus' definition? For marrying Nancy? For violating a Christian belief?

Most liberal Christians and Jews accept divorce as part of our Western culture. They do not encourage it, and they officiate at marriages they hope will be lasting, just as the Leaders of the Ethical Culture Movement and counselors in the American Humanist Association do. But there is a social reality to be considered. The scandal of having a divorce in the family, which haunted families fifty years ago, is no longer a problem. Divorce is commonplace, with more than one in every three marriages ending that way. Remarriage is popular. To label all those who violate this extreme teaching of Jesus as "adulterers" is not feasible. The idea is outmoded.

The Pain in Adultery

What few stop to consider is the pain associated with adultery. The woman who discovers that her husband has been carrying on a romance on the side, whether the affair be of short or long standing, is apt to feel betrayed. The vows taken, the associations built, the investment of time and self are somehow stained and rendered less meaningful. The hurt can be deep and abiding. For the man, the experience of the cuckold can be equally devastating. It reflects the devaluation of the old double-standard of morality, where it was understood that a man might, with impunity, carry on an affair on the side without neglecting or harming his marriage. Now the private domain of the male has been invaded and the result is often anger mingled with fear and shame. Somehow he has failed to be man enough to hold "his woman," and his territorial boundaries have been violated.

For a long time women have been encouraged to be forgiving and understanding wives. They have learned that the "affair" was a short-term fling and that the man had no intention of breaking up the family. Now the male is learning that in many cases the woman never imagined breaking up her marriage, that the affair was short-term, and that she deeply loves and cares about her husband.

Therapists have often been able to help couples move beyond the anger, hurt, and deep pain of adultery. The ability to put the past in the past is difficult but not impossible. Much depends on the depth of the love that unites the two persons; much depends on the forgiving spirit in each; much depends upon the skill of the therapist.

Where the marriage is on the boring level—like that of the Robinsons in the film *The Graduate*, it may be possible for a bored wife (or a bored husband) to carry on secret assignations without ever touching anything that exists in the marriage. Some couples who care about each other give each other permission for discreet affairs that are never talked about. Experience with couples in such alliances has indicated that often the arrangement is really not very satisfactory and that the marriage is close to collapse.

Couples who live together in a marriagelike relationship, but one not based on formal vows, experience the same pain, anger, confusion, and doubt as married couples do when their relationship is intruded upon by one partner finding another bed-companion. Here, because no legal documents have been signed, it is easier for one person to pack up and leave. Often the couple have been together for a relatively short period of time and the mutual investment in property, housing, and so on, is minimal. The pain at discovering the "adulterous" behavior of such a partner is no less devastating than it is among married couples.

NOTES

1. Demetrios J. Constantelos, *The Greek Orthodox Church: Faith, History and Practice* (New York, 1967), p. 87.

2. N. G. M. Van Doornik, S. Jelsma, A. Van de Lisdonk, *A Handbook of the Catholic Faith* (New York, 1956, 1962), p. 335.

15

Incest

As far back as we are able to go in the study of human behavior we find prohibitions against sex or marriage between close relatives. Violation of these restrictions is incest. The details of the rules vary, but most forbid sex between siblings, between parents, and between their children and grandchildren.

In ancient Mesopotamia, laws that were believed to be given by the gods forbade incest. At the same time, in Mesopotamian myths the gods engaged in incestuous behavior. In one myth, a father god impregnated both his daughter and grand-daughter and there was no condemnation of his behavior.[1] In another one, a goddess and her son engage in sexual relations, after which the son murders his father and copulates with his sister.[2]

The Hammurabi code (1728–1626 B.C.E.) outlawed intercourse between a father and his daughter or daughter-in-law and between a mother or foster mother and her son. Penalties for violations varied but included exile, disinheritance, and death.[3] What was permissible for the gods was not permissible for humans. There was one behavior code for divine beings and another for human beings. Whether or not this discrepancy in behavior patterns ever troubled the people of Mesopotamia is not known. It was accepted that the gods had powers and privileges (including immortality) not available to humankind; what gods could do, people could not do. The gods gave the laws; their worshipers were destined to obey.

In Egypt a different social pattern prevailed. Incestuous marriages were acceptable on both the divine and human levels. Geb, the earth god, and Nut, his twin sister, the sky goddess, were parents of Isis and Osiris, who were husband and wife, and of Set and Nephthys, who were also paired. The ithyphallic god Min, who is always portrayed with an erection and who was sometimes called "the bull of his mother," was saluted in the harvest festival with the cry: "Hail Min, who impregnated his mother! How mysterious is that which you have done to her in the darkness."[4]

Incestuous marriage in ancient Egypt was linked to the way in which power and property were transmitted within families. Although the male was the master of the

91

family estates, when his wife died, by Egyptian custom control of the property passed to the eldest daughter. To protect his interests and to keep the property within the family, a father would marry his daughter or a brother would marry his sister. Should the daughter marry outside of her family, the property would be controlled by her husband and hence would be linked to his family and its estates.[5]

In ancient Canaan, sexual encounters are recorded between the fertility god Ba'al and his sister Anat. At this moment it is not known whether incestuous marriages were allowed in Canaanite society or what limits were placed on marriage with near or far family members.

In other cultures throughout the world incestuous relationships have been allowed as part of certain specific tribal rituals. In an African tribe living along the Nkotami River, incest is condoned as part of the ritual of preparation for the hunt. Among some Indians of the Sierra Madre mountains in Mexico, incest is linked to economic benefits. The Kalangs of Java utilize incest as a magical inducement of prosperity. In some groups the practice represents the way life has always been.[6]

Most incest prohibitions forbid intermarriage between blood relatives, but definitions of "blood relatives" differ and thus regulations vary from group to group. Where incestuous marriages are outlawed, sex with near-relatives is also forbidden.

Biblical laws forbidding intermarriage or sex with near-relatives resemble the regulations of Mesopotamia rather than the practices of Egypt. In addition, the Bible records several folk tales about incest, without passing judgment on the act or the participants. One such story concerns the patriarch Abraham and his wife Sarah.

This particular story of Abraham and Sarah is one of three variations on the same theme: the attempt to pass off one's wife as a sister. The idea behind the narratives is that the woman is so beautiful that, if it were known she were married, her suitors would murder her husband so that she would be a widow and eligible for remarriage. To protect her husband, the woman pretends to be her husband's sister.

The oldest of the accounts is about Isaac and Rebekah in Gerar (Gen. 26:1–33). Isaac pretended that Rebekah was his sister, but King Abimelech observed Isaac petting (*tsahak*) with Rebekah and commented that this was not the sort of behavior a man ordinarily engaged in with his sister. Isaac admitted the deceptions. A similar story is recorded about Abraham and Sarah in Egypt. In this account Sarah actually became part of Pharaoh's harem before the deception was discovered (Gen. 12:10–20). In the third version, Abraham and Sarah were in Gerar, and the king (as in the Isaac and Rebekah account) was Abimelech (Gen. 20). Sarah, as Abraham's sister, actually ended up in bed with Abimelech. Before any sexual encounter took place, the deity intervened and saved Sarah from becoming involved in a sexual encounter with the king. The editor explained Abraham's deception by having the patriarch explain that Sarah was indeed his half-sister. They both had the same father, but different mothers. There is no criticism of this incestuous marriage or of the deception.

Another incestuous legend involves Lot, Abraham's nephew, and Lot's daughter. The setting for the tale is the area not far from the cities of Sodom and Gomorrah. Lot's wife had been turned into a pillar of salt because she had disobeyed Yahweh and "looked back." Lot and his two daughters took refuge in a cave. The account reads as follows:

And he [Lot] lived with his two daughters in a cave. The elder said to the younger, "Our father is getting old, there is not a man left on earth to mate with us as the custom was throughout the world. Come let us intoxicate our father with wine, then we will have intercourse with him so we may keep our seed alive through our father." That night, after they had intoxicated their father with wine, the elder one went in and had intercourse with her father; he was unaware of her coming and going. The next day, the elder said to the younger, "See, last night I copulated with our father. Tonight let's intoxicate him again with wine, and you go in and have intercourse with him so that we may keep our seed alive through him." So after they had intoxicated their father with wine, the younger went in and had intercourse with him and he was not aware of her coming or going. So it happened that both of Lot's daughters became pregnant by their father. The elder bore a son whom she named Moab ("from father") and he is the progenitor of the Moabites of today. The younger also bore a son whom she named Ben-Ammi ("son of my people"); he is the father of the Ammonites of today. [Gen. 19:30–38]

Incest is not condemned in the story. Indeed the tale may be related to an older myth of divine destruction of the universe—a kind of substitute flood myth. The eldest daughter complained that there were no men left on earth with whom she might procreate. Whatever the earlier history of the account might have been, in its present setting it is a folk tale. As a folk tale it may have been designed to explain the feeling of family connection between the Hebrews and their Ammonite and Moabite neighbors. It might also have been designed to denigrate these neighboring peoples as offsprings of incestuous relations and therefore not quite up to the purer ancestral lines of the Hebrews. If this fragment of folk fiction is nothing more than a putdown of Moabites and Ammonites, it can be said to support the idea that incest, even under the extreme conditions of isolation in a cave, still comes under subtle reproach and condemnation.

Another folk tale about incest involves a concubine. Although concubines were not given the same status as wives in the Hebrew household, they were considered to be part of the extended family and might even have been considered possessions. In any case, they came under the same kind of protection against incest as any other member of the family, and having intercourse with the concubine belonging to one's father was tantamount to violation of the incest taboo. Jacob, who is called "Israel" in some passages, had a concubine named Bilhah. His son Reuben copulated with her. The truncated account does not record what Israel's (Jacob's) reactions were and states only that the father "heard of it" (Gen. 35:22). In a subsequent passage Reuben was cursed by his father and lost his privileged status as first-born son. His tribe is condemned to increasing weakness because their progenitor "defiled" his father's bed (Gen. 49:3; cf. 1 Chron. 5:1). The story appears to have been developed when the Reubenites were diminishing in numbers; the folk tale explains why.

One biblical account that appears to have a basis in fact is recorded in the court history of King David. David's son Absalom rebelled against his father and in the struggle that ensued drove his father from the throne in Jerusalem. As he departed, David left ten concubines, members of his royal harem, to care for the palace (2 Sam. 15:16). When Absalom occupied the city, he pitched his tent on the palace roof, where he could be observed by all of the inhabitants of Jerusalem. He then publicly sexually possessed the members of his father's harem. The act was more than a statement of defiance; it signified that he had taken his father's place and that he was now master of the palace and ruler of the kingdom. David had done exactly the same thing when he replaced King Saul; he had sexually possessed Saul's wives (2 Sam. 12:8). The same principle was involved when Saul's commander, Abner, wished to take over Saul's kingdom from Saul's son Ishbosheth. He possessed Saul's concubine Rizpah. When he was called to account for this act, he reacted in fury and betrayed his king (2 Sam. 3:6–21). Later, when Adonijah petitioned Solomon for their father's (King David's) last bed partner, Abishag the Shunnamite, it cost Adonijah his life; for Solomon was aware that his brother was making a bid for the crown. Thus the incestuous act by Absalom was in actuality a political statement, a social act to demonstrate his authority. When David regained control of his throne and palace, he isolated the concubines and denied them any sexual relationships, because they had been made unclean or unfit through Absalom's act (2 Sam. 20:3).

Biblical laws prohibiting incest are explicit. Leviticus 18 is part of what scholars have labeled the "Holiness code," because it lays down the rules that must be obeyed if Israel is to be a "holy" people acceptable to their god Yahweh. The code was formulated during the sixth century, when the nation was in exile in Babylon; but there can be no doubt that materials from earlier periods were reworked and incorporated.

The code stipulated that the way of Israel was not to be the way of Canaan or Egypt: "You shall not do as they do in Egypt where you lived, and you shall not do as they do in Canaan . . . you shall not conform to their customs" (Lev. 18:3). Hebrew law forbade an individual to have intercourse with either parent, a sister, a niece or nephew, an aunt, uncle, daughter or daughter-in-law, a sister-in-law, or a grandchild. Because children could be the offspring of a single father but a different mother, the laws exclude sexual relations with any blood relative, although marriage to a half-sister was permissible at certain times (cf. Gen. 20:12; 2 Sam. 13:7–13).

The penalties for violation of the incest laws ranged from excommunication to the threat of being cursed with childlessness to death. A cursing ritual composed during the Babylonian exile (sixth century B.C.E.) is recorded in Deuteronomy 27. A man who copulates with his father's wife or with a sister or half-sister is cursed. How these punishments were carried out is not recorded.

The very fact that legislation was needed to prohibit incestuous sex implies that it was not uncommon among the Hebrew people. Indeed the prophet Ezekiel, who wrote from Babylon during the sixth century B.C.E., scathingly denounced the people of Jerusalem. Among his indictments were the sexual relationships between a father and a daughter-in-law and between brother and sister (Ezek. 22:11).

In modern times, laws prohibiting marriage or sex between close relatives vary from place to place. Prohibitions against uncle-niece, aunt-nephew, and first-cousin marriages and intercourse are common, but are accepted in some communities depending upon whether the kinship lines are maternal or paternal. Some groups bar intermarriage or sex between step-relatives and members of the same family who are adoptees. Marriage and coitus between close relatives who have been separated at birth and who later meet and fall in love are not only the stuff of myths (Oedipus) and fiction (Henry Fielding's *The Life and History of Tom Jones, a Foundling*) but occur often in modern lives that sometimes make the news.

Modern prohibitions were no doubt influenced indirectly by the almost universal taboos against intermarriage with blood relatives, but probably more directly by biblical teachings. Some endorsement of the wisdom of this taboo has come from an awareness of the biological factors that may be involved. Modern studies have indicated that there are higher incidents of mental retardation and congenital defects resulting from incestuous marriages. On the other hand, as cattle breeders can tell us, it is possible that, out of the animal breeding of father-daughter and mother-son, desired strengths can be enhanced. However, biologists and sociologists point out that human groups that insist on out-breeding rather than in-breeding are favored and preserved by the process of the survival of the fittest.

There are numerous speculative theories about why the incest taboo is so widespread. It has been suggested that the taboo protects the patterns of authority and status in the family. Love relations with pregnancies between a parent and child could raise problems with traditional responsibilities of childrearing or with the household responsibilities of the adults. Sibling intimacies and pregnancies might divide the family, causing alliances of children against parents. Because fathers tend to ''fall in love with'' their daughters and mothers with their sons (and vice versa) the potentials for jealous anger between the parents and the sexually involved offspring could be divisive. No matter how poor our perception of the origins of the taboos may be or how dimly we may understand why differences in the taboo exist, the reality of the prohibition affects society.

Child Molestation and Incest

There is a special dimension of incestuous relationships that is only beginning to receive the attention it warrants, although it is clear that the problem is as old as time: it is the manipulative incestuous sexual molestation of children by older adults. Many psychologists accept the relationship between pre-adolescent siblings of about the same age who explore one another's bodies and perhaps even engage in coitus as part of the normal process of investigating aspects of human physiology. Usually such engagements are short term, do not involve the manipulation of one child by the other, and are participated in by mutual consent. Socially healthy children do not linger over this phase of their probing of life; they move on to other areas of inquiry. It is when the relationship is ongoing, having developed out of the manipulation of a younger child by an older sibling, that pathological dimensions become apparent.

Sometimes older sisters begin their exploration of sex with a younger brother. Away from the family, where they feel safe, they caress the child to erection and may even experiment with intromission. They guarantee his silence with bribes of candy or with threats to reveal some bad thing he has done. More often it is an older brother who imposes his will on the younger sister, by engaging her in a game of "playing house" or "playing grownup." Because the younger child loves and respects her brother, she cooperates, despite the confused feelings of being involved in behavior that does not feel right or good. Sometimes the older sibling uses threats or other manipulating techniques to control the situation. Whenever the older brother manipulates the younger sister into incestuous behavior, some damage is done to the girl.

Parent-child sexual relations are more common. For example, a father estranged from his wife enters into a sexual relationship with the oldest daughter. When she leaves the home, he may turn his attention to the next daughter. In some instances there is evidence of an unarticulated conspiracy between father, mother, and daughter. The daughter is the victim. She is too young to protect herself—molestation can begin when the child is five or six years old and extend through puberty into the late teens and beyond. She is bound by love and loyalty to her parents, upon whom she is dependent for support and existence. She feels she has no one to complain to. When she tries to tell her mother, her statements are ignored. She is told by her father that, if anyone outside of the family should learn of the relationship, she could be responsible for the breakup of the family, that she and her brothers or sisters, if there are any, would be placed in foster homes and the father would go to jail, leaving no one to support the mother. She is terrified of desertion and abandonment. The guilt of being responsible for the demolition of the family is more than she can contemplate bearing. Her natural feelings of love for her father have become confused because of his physical invasion of her body. She is torn and bewildered. She is alone. She is a victim.

Sometimes the incest begins after the mother or the father dies. The daughter or the son becomes the replacement for the dead mate, and the parent receives from the child all the physical and some of the domestic services previously provided by the spouse. Often these households tend to be isolated, with little contact with outsiders. In some instances an angry or perhaps a drunken father beats both wife and daughter into submission and, by terrorizing them, maintains sexual control of both.

Some psychologists have suggested that in most cases no real harm has been done to the child by the sexual experience. The evidence suggests something else. Disturbed behavior-patterns in the adult have been traced directly to incestuous experiences. The wife who becomes cold and unresponsive when her husband reaches the age of forty-five may have been molested by her father or some other male relative when he was at that age. She may protest that it only happened once or twice or three times, but the impact on the psyche is profound. The secrecy that surrounds the sexual act is toxic and guilt-producing. The need to mentally deny the reality of what happened or to suppress the memory of the violation is burdensome. The confusion of the child who does not really understand her body responses and who cannot comprehend what is happening to her remains as an unresolved conflict of emotions and feelings. Extensive therapy is required to alleviate the feelings that continue to cling in the mind—the feelings of unworthiness, of betrayal, and of having been violated.

Similar response patterns appear when an older sibling molests a younger sister or brother, or when the molester is the mother and the victim is the son, or when the molestation is homosexual. The victim is reduced to a sexual object and is made to feel worthless, unimportant, and unclean. It is not surprising to find that some molested women become whores—after all, they have been made to feel that they are not worth much, and certainly not worthy of the love that is associated with stable marriage relations. Susan Forward and Craig Buck have expressed the issue in the following terms:

> Incest is powerful. Its devastation is greater than that of nonincestuous child molestation or rape because incest is set within a constellation of family emotions and conflicts. There is no stranger to run from, no home to run to. The child cannot feel safe in his or her own bed. The victim must learn to live with incest; it flavors the child's entire world. The aggressor is always there. Incest is often a continuing horror for the victim.   .   .   . Think of the lowest thing in the world, and whatever it is, I'm lower.[7]

There are some of us who can only feel annoyance and anger when we read or hear the comment that the child probably enjoyed the experience and perhaps had even asked for it! The implication is that little girls are not always all that innocent and may actually provoke intimacies, an attitude that seems to go back to the interpretation of the Garden of Eden myth, with Eve as the temptress of Adam. One mother commented that her four-year-old daughter was a "flirt," fluttering her eyelashes at men, wiggling her hips provocatively, thrusting her pelvis forward in what appeared to be a mock sexual gesture and engaging in extensive kissing and hugging of males. The mother implied that her daughter's innate sexual instincts were surfacing at an early age and suggested that she would be involved with some boy by the time "she is six."

No one will argue that human sexual responses are not inborn. Little boys are often born with an erection and children find their genitals and experience genital pleasure early in life. But sexual behavior patterns are learned. The little girl was copying behavior she had observed—perhaps in the antics of neighboring teen-agers, perhaps as she watched her mother flirt with her father, perhaps on the television screen—somewhere she learned that this is the way a woman (girl) behaves toward males. Perhaps the mature male bird comes naturally to the mating dance by which he hopes to persuade the female, who performs her own fluttering response, to become his mate. But all little children do not engage in the sexual behavior of this particular child and it is to be doubted that she had any understanding of her tiny body and its sexual functions. She learned flirtation as a way of coping with older people. The males responded, and her mother thought she was "cute." Children are intuitive, they learn early what "games" impress adults and win approval.

No doubt the *Lolita* story educated many to think that some little girls simply accept sexual intercourse as a manipulative tool and that no real harm is done to the child. The child got the rewards she sought, the man was sexually satisfied, so who was hurt? It is also a fact that during incestuous intercourse some girls do experience orgasms, and orgasmic responses are pleasure responses; but because the orgasmic response during incest is mingled with a medley of other feelings, most of which are negative, toxic, and confusing, the use of the word "pleasure" in this context seems absolutely inappropriate. The older individual who uses a child for his or her own sexual gratification is not really interested in what the child is feeling; the adult cares only for his or her own promiscuous sexual feelings. It is only recently that awareness of the traumatic damage done to the psyche of the child has surfaced.

Information about incestuous molestation is limited at present and is only slowly emerging. Incest is a closet subject. Many adults are unwilling to talk about their childhood experiences; they prefer to try to forget the whole affair. Children are intimidated into silence. But breakthroughs are occurring. Adults are becoming aware that relational problems in later life can be traced to traumatic childhood experiences. In group settings they feel free to share what happened to them with others who can listen with the understanding of someone who "has been there." The help of a trained therapist enables individuals to cope with what has happened to them.

Prosecution of parents who molest children falters in many states. To imprison the father and break up the family or to remove the child and place him or her in a foster home appear to be drastic measures to some. Nevertheless, social workers and jurists who have become aware of the damage done by incestuous molestation and manipulation and who are committed to the protection of the child realize that without such measures the child is in danger of moving back into a destructive environment. Therapy for the parents and the child, and in many cases for the whole family and even an extended family, are important for healing interfamily relationships and the wounds to the psyche.

There is a recidivistic dimension in incest that troubles therapists and there is solid evidence that many molesters of members of their own family will repeat their behavior on another sibling or on one of their own children or grandchildren. By exposing the pathological behavior to members of the family, parents can be warned to protect their children from the molester and to avoid providing opportunities for molestation. Families can encourage children not to let themselves be touched on the genitals or breasts by older persons and to report any violations.

Perhaps Sirach, the wise Jew, was aware of the burning sexual demands of one who engages in incestuous behavior when he wrote:

> A man who fornicates with his near kin ["fornicator with the body of his flesh"] will in no way stop until he has kindled a fire (or "until he has been consumed by fire"). [Sirach 23:16]

Child Molestation in the Bible

There is only one possible reference to sibling molestation in the Bible, and the situation is so vague that molestation may not be involved. Some interpreters have suggested that the reason Sarah demanded that her handmaid Hagar and Ishmael, Hagar's son by Abraham, be expelled from the family was because Sarah saw Ishmael masturbating Isaac.

The setting for the story is the festive occasion marking the weaning of Isaac, who would have been three or four years old at that time. Ishmael would be about fifteen. The passage reads:

> Sarah noticed that the son whom Hagar, the Egyptian, had born to Abraham was playing with her son Isaac. [Gen. 21:9]

The last four words are missing from the Hebrew text but are found in the Greek (Septuagint) and Latin (Vulgate) versions. The Hebrew verb *tzahak* is clearly a wordplay on the name Isaac (*yitzak*), and it can mean "to laugh with" as well as "to fondle sexually," as it does in the story about Rebecca and Isaac fondling each other in Gerar (Gen. 26:8). Some commentators have suggested that Ishmael was only amusing the infant Isaac and that Sarah's hostility was nothing more than a mother's jealousy. Others think that reference is to the molestation of a child by a teen-aged step-brother that provoked Sarah's reaction. Expulsion because of jealousy seems too harsh; expulsion because of molestation seems more natural. No matter how one interprets the story, the results were the same: Hagar and Ishmael were sent away.

The Hawk and the Chicken (or Dove)

Older males who prey sexually upon young children are known as "hawks." They often have a long history of child molestation and generally have feelings of deep insecurity about sex with adults. They do not fall into any age group and their behavior can extend from early childhood into old age. The hawk is a "loner" who has learned to identify potential victims—children who feel isolated and estranged, children who hunger for attention and friendship. The hawk can recognize these "chickens" in places as public as the shopping mall. He approaches the child with some word of appreciation. The girl has pretty hair, eyes, or hands. The boy is a fine looking fellow. If he gets a response, he moves into the next phase of friendship-building and asks questions. Where are the parents? What are they doing? He offers them candy, or invites them to a theater, or offers to walk with them. Some single out a neighborhood boy who lives with a divorced mother. The hawk becomes a "substitute" father, "an older brother," and wins the support of the mother who encourages her son to go to the ballgame with the neighbor, who is perhaps only ten years older than her son. Before long, the child is involved in sexual relations with a person he or she has come to love and care about. To complain or inform is to lose a friendship that pays off in attention, gifts, and feelings of worth.

Hawks often limit their interest to children of a certain age group. A boy of nine or ten is just right for one "hawk," and when he becomes eleven he is discarded for a new, younger chicken. Another prefers the fourteen- or fifteen-year-old. Little girls of ten or eleven fascinate another. Once the child passes the desirable age he or she is replaced.

Some hawks use children for pornographic purposes. The children are photographed in the nude, masturbating, or engaging in sex with the "hawk" (whose face is not shown) or with another child. There is a lucrative business in "child porn," and it thrives on the abuse of children.

When the perpetrators of sexual crimes against children are arrested and sentenced, they are despised by other prisoners. It is a common assumption that any new convict who enters the prison carrying a Bible is probably a child molester. Prison officials know that he will be in constant danger of attack from other convicts, even those whose crime might appear to be equally serious (rape, homicide, and so on). There is something about the sexual abuse of a child that produces feelings of disgust, anger, and repugnance in the prisoners. It may stem from the knowledge that child-molesters are weak people who feel they must control the sex object and who are only comfortable with children. It may arise out of the awareness that child molesters often continue to deny their offense and, when released, repeat it—they do not change because of punishment. Perhaps it is the piousity that is associated with so many molesters. These psychopathic individuals are alone and friendless within the prison walls and without. More and more sentences include the provision for extensive psychotherapy for hawks.

The religious affectation of the hawk does not in any way imply that any modern religious group endorses or supports or affirms his behavior. Religious leaders and members of faith groups are appalled by the molestation of children, just as any decent person is. Most are aware that the hawk is a psychopathic personality who may himself have been the victim of molestation. Despite feelings of outrage, Jews and Christians, as well as other groups, encourage therapy for the hawk and the victimized child and try to find ways to protect children from molestation. Some churches provide space for concerned parents and others to meet; some introduce the subject in parochial meetings and in sermons. All have deep concerns.

NOTES

1. "Enki and Ninhursag: A Paradise Myth," *ANET*, pp. 37–40.

2. "A Babylonia Theogony," *ANET*, pp. 517 f.

3. "The Code of Hammurabi," laws 154–158, *ANET*.

4. E. O. James, *Seasonal Feasts and Festivals* (New York, 1961) p. 53.

5. Cf. Margaret Murray, *The Splendor that was Egypt.* (New York, 1963) pp. 100 ff.

6. For a brief summary, see Susan Forward and Craig Buck, *Betrayal of Innocence* (New York, 1979), pp. 9–12. For a detailed study, see William Graham Sumner, *Folkways: A Study of the Sociological Importance of Usages* (New York, 1940).

7. Forward and Buck, op. cit., p. 19.

16

Rape

When biblical writers describe rape they tell of the man seizing (*tapash*) a woman or overpowering (*hezik*) her before copulating with her. The Deuteronomic law reads:

> If a man meets a young woman, a virgin who is not betrothed, and he seizes [*tapash*] her and copulates with her and they are discovered, the man who copulated with her must pay to the father of the young woman fifty shekels of silver and she shall be his wife, because he debased [*inna*] her he may not divorce her throughout his life. [Deut. 22:28–29]

> If a man meets a betrothed young woman in the open country and the man overpowers [*hezik*] her and copulates with her; then only the man who copulated with her shall die. Nothing shall be done to the young woman, there is no death-evil in the young woman. [Deut. 22:25–26]

In both cases the male uses strength to overcome any resistance the woman might offer. In the second, because the man raped the woman in the open country, away from possible rescue, only he is liable. She is the recognized victim. If the rape had occurred within the town or city, both would have been stoned to death; the assumption being that the woman could have cried out for help. The fact that she was raped in a setting where help may have been forthcoming determined that she was a willing participant (Deut. 22:23–24). The man who raped a betrothed woman in the open country and the man who raped in the city were both killed, because they violated a woman belonging to another man. The woman raped in the city was killed because she let it happen.

The first law provides for the payment of the bridal price to the girl's father. He gets the money due to him. He gets a son-in-law, and the daughter gets a husband (albeit a rapist)—all proper procedure within the Hebrew idea of marriage and family. Because betrothal was considered to be the equivalent of marriage, perhaps the woman raped in the field would be able to marry her fiancé.

No reference is made to the feelings of the woman. In each instance she is treated very much as a possession. To despoil the property of another man is to break Hebrew law and be subject to punishment. If the male who controls the woman is the father, the rapist pays the bridal fee; if the controlling party is her betrothed, the rapist is killed.

A legend recounts the rape of Dinah, the daughter of Jacob and Leah, by the uncircumcised Prince Shechem, who "saw her, siezed [*laqah*] her, copulated with her and debased [*inna*] her" (Gen. 34:2), after which he longed for her and wanted to marry her. His father, Hamor, approached Jacob to make marriage arrangements that would be in accord with the Deuteronomic law cited above. But Dinah's brothers were determined to avenge the family honor and remove the stain of the serious sexual offense (*nebala*), which affected the entire community. They insisted that, if the families were to be united, the men of Hamor's community, including, of course, Shechem, must be circumcised. An agreement was reached, but when the circumcised men were still sore from the operation, Dinah's brothers murdered all the males and took everything in the city as booty, including the slain men's wives. No reference is made to Dinah's feelings, or to the feelings of the captive women.

When the men of Gibeah sought to sexually possess the Levite visiting in their town, he gave them his concubine to be used in their lust (Judg. 19). She was a victim of gang rape (the Hebrew term *alal* means "abuse" or "use wantonly"). Their vicious act resulted in a civil war in which an army composed of a confederation of Hebrew tribes wiped out all but six hundred men of the tribe of Benjamin, of which the Gibeahite rapists were a part. Then the Hebrews felt they may have overreacted to the gang rape. They met to decide what to do with the remaining six hundred Benjaminites. They had vowed to Yahweh that they would never give their daughters to any Benjaminites for marriage; but unless the six hundred found wives the whole tribe would disappear. On the other hand, they dared not violate the oath they had sworn to Yahweh, lest he turn against them. They decided to out-maneuver the deity; they would keep the letter of the vow, but not the spirit. They sent word to the men of Benjamin that their daughters would perform the annual vineyard dance at Shiloh. They suggested that, while the young women were dancing through the grape arbors, the men of Benjamin swoop down and seize (*hataph*: carry off by force) the young women, who would become their wives (Judg. 20–21). Gang rape resulted in warfare that ended with planned mass rape.

David's son Amnon raped his half-sister Tamar. The young prince was so overcome by desire for his young sister that he actually became ill. He used his illness as an opportunity to entrap the young woman. He asked King David to have Tamar prepare food and bring it to him. When she brought the food he overpowered (*hazek*) her and said, "Copulate with me, my sister" (2 Sam. 13:11). She protested and told him to ask David for her hand in marriage. He refused and "overpowered [*hezak*] her and debased [*inna*] her and copulated with her"

(13:14). Having raped her, he then despised her. She suffered a double loss: the loss of her virginity, which was of prime importance in ancient Israel, and the loss of the respect of her brother. The rejection was the greater burden (13:16). Because she had been violated, she went into mourning, tearing the distinctive garment that was worn by virgins in ancient Israel, putting ashes on her head (a sign of grief), and weeping. Although David was angry over Amnon's behavior he took no action; but Tamar's brother Absalom finally revenged the incestuous rape of his sister by killing Amnon (13:28 f.). Here, for the first time, the writer, who appears to have been a sensitive historian, recorded the feelings of the violated woman. But the story of Tamar stops with her immediate grief. There is no record of her subsequent reactions to what could only have been a devastating experience. The death of Amnon put the scale of Israelite justice in balance, so to speak, but the pain experienced by the woman was not considered worthy of further record.

When Hebrew soldiers went to war and captured a city, they did what victors have done in wars throughout history—they plundered the city. Included in the booty were the women, who as prizes of war could become slaves in their captors' homes and certainly were used for sexual gratification by the men. Indeed, the laws of Deuteronomy provide for the taking of women and children as booty (Deut. 20:14), but the regulations in Numbers 31:17–18 call for the preservation of virgins only, whom the men may keep for themselves. One can only assume that the terrified women had no choice but to submit sexually to the soldiers who became their masters.

One cannot help but wonder to what extent the biblical attitude toward rape and rape victims has affected present-day attitudes. Concern for the woman and her feelings is not a primary concern in the biblical laws and narratives. What really matters in each account, except perhaps in the story of Tamar, is the effect of the rape on the family reputation or status, the loss of virginity for which payment is made to the woman's father, and the proper punishment for the rapist. The woman is an object. Only in the Tamar account does the historian, who may have been very close to the event, permit us to be aware of the young woman's pain.

The False Accusation

A patriarchal legend relates that, when Joseph as a young man was in Egypt working as a personal slave in the household of one of Pharaoh's eunuchs named Potiphar, he was falsely accused of rape (Gen. 39). The account notes that Joseph was handsome and that Potiphar's wife "lifted her eyes at" (gave the eye to?) him and said, "Lie [have sex] with me." Joseph refused and reminded the woman of his loyalty to Potiphar, of the fact that she was a married woman, and of his refusal to violate a divine law. She was not dissuaded, but day after day continued her provocative cajoling, until one day, in frustration, she seized his cloak and demanded "Lie [have sex] with me!" Joseph ran away but left his cloak behind. The angry woman called the servants and said "Look, he [her husband] had to import this Hebrew person to fondle [*tsahak*] us! He burst in upon me to lie [have sex] with me, but when I screamed loudly [lifted my voice and called], he fled leaving his cloak with me." When Potiphar came home, she said, "The Hebrew slave that you brought here broke in to fondle me, but when I screamed he dropped his cloak and ran out of the house." Joseph was imprisoned and only later, because of his skill as a dream interpreter, was he released.

There is a close correlation between this story and the Egyptian "Tale of the Two Brothers," upon which the Joseph story may have been based.[1] In the Egyptian story, Bata lived with his older brother Anubis and Anubis's wife. One day Bata was sent back to the house to get seed for sowing the fields. As he entered, Anubis's wife was fixing her hair. She was attracted by Bata's strength and fine figure. She put her arms around him and invited him to spend an hour in sexual intercourse, promising to sew him fine clothes in return. Bata became very angry, so angry he frightened the woman. He told her that she and her husband were like parents to him and that she was inviting him to participate in a "great crime." He told her he wanted the matter dropped and would not tell anyone about it. But she was afraid he might tell. So she ingested fat and grease to make herself vomit, and made herself appear to have been criminally attacked. When her husband came home, she told him that Bata had asked her to spend an hour copulating and had ordered her to put on her wig for the occasion.

The older brother reacted in fury. He hid behind the barn door waiting for Bata, who was coming in with the cattle. Now magical elements begin to appear in the story. Bata's communication with the animals was so good that they warned him of his brother's presence and he fled, pursued by the spear-carrying Anubis. As they ran, the young man prayed to the sun god and the god heard his prayer and caused a lake filled with crocodiles to separate the brothers. From the far side, Bata told Anubis what had really happened, and to underscore his innocence drew a knife and cut off his penis, which he hurled in the lake, where it was eaten by a fish! The brothers were now reconciled and Anubis returned home to kill his wife.

Both the Hebrew story and the Egyptian tale are examples of a motif that is familiar in world literature: the seductive woman who is thwarted in her efforts.[2] Indeed, "Hell has no fury like a woman scorned." Other motifs are also present: the woman as seductress, the unfaithful wife, and masculine honor and loyalty. In each case the man was accused of attempted rape or of actual rape; in each case the man was innocent. Because these ideas have become part of our social thinking, it is not surprising that women who have cried "rape" have not always been heard.

The Modern Setting

In *Webster's Third International Dictionary* (unabridged), rape is defined as "illicit sexual intercourse without the consent of the woman and effected by force, duress, intimidation or deception as to the nature of the act." Until recently this definition did not include the possible rape of a wife by a husband. Sexual intercourse, no matter how obtained and regardless of what force might have been used, was a husband's privilege. This law has been successfully challenged in Oregon. Now, due in large measure to the feminist movement, more attention is being given to forced coitus, particularly in reported cases of battered wives.

Nor have women who reported rape always been well treated in the police precincts or in the courtroom where they faced the accused rapist and his lawyer. Some policemen were not sympathetic; some were halfway convinced that the woman probably "asked for it" or that she may have fabricated the story to get even with a boyfriend with whom she was angry. Some were impatient with her hysteria. In the courtroom, often the victim was harassed by the suspect's lawyer, her past sex behavior was probed, her response during the rape was questioned, and she was asked such brutally demeaning questions as "Did you enjoy the sex?" or "Did you climax?" The image of the woman as the temptress was often accentuated. If she wore clothing that some male might consider "sexy," the rapist's attorney might point out that the woman's intention was to provoke interest from men. Surveys show that many women who dress in attractive or appealing clothing are dressing for themselves—they wear what makes them feel feminine and beautiful—or are following a style. There is no real evidence to demonstrate that they are seeking to attract men. What was most amazing in the rape trials was the absence of emphasis on the lack of control exhibited by the men. It was almost as if it was assumed that certain colors or kinds of dress tempted men and that women were supposed to wear dowdy, unattractive clothes to protect men from themselves! The feminist movement has been a powerful force in changing the response to the rape victim in the police station and in the courtroom. Trained and sensitive female police officers may now interview the woman and see that she gets medical care. Courtroom procedures have been tightened.

Although many rapes are by men who are known to the women they attack, many other rapes are by strangers. In some instances the woman is able to repel the intruder and actually fight him off, despite the difference in physical strength. In other cases, the woman is terrified or threatened with a knife or other weapon and compelled to submit. The fact that there is no evidence of a struggle, no bruises or contusions to demonstrate resistance, has prompted some investigators to assume that the woman must have cooperated willingly. Classes in self-defense help some women overcome the social conditioning that has tended to make them nonphysical and nonviolent. They learn to overcome terror, muster physical resources, and fight back. Some carry weapons to protect themselves.

Attention has been given to the post-rape syndrome. Immediately after the rape, many women are completely disoriented. It seems unbelievable to them that they have been violated. They are too shaken to be hysterical or too hysterical to know what to do. They feel soiled and may take a shower to remove the filth that they feel has been inflicted on them—and by doing so they destroy important evidence. Mental anguish may produce nausea, trembling, sobbing, and physical weakness. Later they may be troubled by nightmares and be irritable, be unable to focus or concentrate, and may have little interest in food. Once past the traumatic shock, they may make dramatic changes in life-style. They may move to another city or state and sever relations with friends of long standing because they feel no one really understands what they have experienced. They may withdraw from any association with males or experience dis-ease in the company of men or develop morbid fears of men who bear even the slightest physical resemblance to the rapist. Their personal life can suffer. They may experience impaired responses in lovemaking. Marital relations are often strained, and sometimes the husband rejects the woman because she was raped by another man, which can only add feelings of abandonment to the emotional burdens she is already carrying. She may be troubled by flashbacks that recur for years. Rape has both immediate and long-range impact on the victim, and extensive therapy may be required to help repair some of the damage.

Statutory rape is usually defined as coitus with a consenting female who not only is not the man's spouse but who by law is considered too young to be considered mentally competent or mature enough to make decisions of responsible consent. The fact that the woman may have seduced the man is immaterial; only the legal age is a factor, and that may vary from sixteen to eighteen. The National Organization for Women advocates lowering the age of consent to twelve. Most courts distinguish between forcible rape and statutory rape and, by considering the latter unlawful sexual intercourse, punish the man less severely than in rape. When both participants are under the legal age and both are consenting participants, the charge may be changed to delinquency. The age disparity is always an important factor, and the penalty for an older person convicted of statutory rape is always more severe.

All religious organizations condemn rape and the rapist. Few have provisions to care for the emotional needs of the victims or to cope with the pathology of the rapist. Most congregations are deeply concerned with providing proper protection for women against potential rapists, but few have any awareness of the depth of trauma associated with being raped or of the hostility and anger toward women being expressed by the rapist.

The demeaning of women by biblical writers and the general indifference to the feelings of women who have been violated may contribute to the low level of awareness in well-meaning church members who look to the Bible for guidance. The need for extended therapy provided by trained therapists for women who have experienced rape should be emphasized in every congregation. In addition, deep concern for providing adequate help for the rapist is also imperative.

NOTES

1. *ANET*, "The Story of Two Brothers" pp. 23 ff.
2. Theodor H. Gaster, *Myth, Legend and Custom in the Old Testament* (New York, 1969), p. 217.

17

Bestiality

Laws come into being to control situations that already exist. Hebrew regulations against intercourse with animals indicate that there were those who engaged in such acts. The regulations read as follows:

Whoever lies with [has intercourse with] an animal shall be put to death. [Exodus 22:19]

You shall not lie with [copulate with] an animal and pollute yourself with it; nor shall a woman stand before [assume a posture with] an animal to lie with [copulate with] it, it is an abomination. [Lev. 18:23]

And if a man lies carnally [has sex with] an animal he shall be put to death and you shall kill the animal; and if a woman approach [sexually] any animal to copulate with it, you shall kill the woman and the beast, they shall be put to death and their blood is on them. [Lev. 20:15–16]

Cursed is anyone who lies with any animal. [Deut. 27:21].

The intent of the rulings is clear: anyone, man or woman, who engages in sexual relations with an animal is to be killed. In Leviticus 20:15, the animal is also presumed to be guilty and is killed. The Deuteronomic statement is one from a series of ritual curses pronounced by Levites and sanctioned by the community.

The Hittites had laws prohibiting sexual intercourse with pigs, cows, and sheep. The penalty, unless revoked by the monarch, was death. Copulation with a horse or mule was sanctioned.[1] The Canaanite texts found at Ras es-Shamra (Ugarit) contain myths in which the fertility god Ba'al copulates with a heifer:

. . . he [Ba'al] copulates with a heifer in the pasture, with a calf in the field,
he copulates with it seventy-seven times
mounts it eighty-eight times
it conceives and bears . . .[2]

Ritual drama consists of the enactment of the acts of a god or goddess. For example, Passover is celebrated symbolically in present-day Jewish communities; but in a far more literal fashion by Samaritans on Mount Gerazim, where the paschal animals are slaughtered and their blood is smeared on the faces of the participants. Easter is dramatized symbolically in church services, but with greater excitement and fire at the Church of the Holy Sepulchre in Jerusalem. It is therefore quite possible that some dramatization of the myth of the divine impregnation of the heifer by the god Ba'al was enacted at Canaanite shrines in ancient Palestine. The priest might actually mount a heifer or the myth could be symbolically dramatized. The bull was an important image in Canaanite worship and could represent the father god El or the fertility god Ba'al. If real animals were not used, molded replicas might be.

In one story in the collection of Elijah legends, Yahweh told the prophet that he would spare in Israel the seven thousand ''knees that have not genuflected to Ba'al, and each mouth that has not kissed him'' (1 Kings 19:18). Genuflection might refer to the limping ritual dance associated with the worship of Ba'al, a dance referred to in another Elijah legend of a contest between the prophet and the priests of Ba'al on Mount Carmel (1 Kings 18:26). It may also indicate the devout posture of a petitioner or worshiper bowed on one knee before the god—a posture represented in Babylonian and Egyptian sculpture.

The kissing of the god could refer to the acts of worshipers before images of the god similar to those found in the excavations at Ras es-Shamra. It could also point to a ritual in which the figure of the god in the form of a bull was kissed. The kissing of artifacts or symbols is still in vogue in religious ceremonies. Muslims kiss the Ka'aba stone, Jews kiss their fingers and transfer the kiss to the mezuzah as they leave their homes, some Protestants kiss their Bibles, and Roman Catholics kiss the papal ring. The well-worn artifacts of the past indicate the custom has had a long history. It is possible that the reference in the Elijah legend is to a rite of kissing a statue.

In his denunciation of the Ba'al cult, the prophet Hosea referred to craftsmen who molded images for worship and then scornfully added: ''Men kiss calves!'' (Hos. 13:2). It must be admitted that this is a difficult text, but it would appear that Hosea had in mind the cult of the golden calf and the presence of the golden calves in the Hebrew shrines for Yahweh at Dan and Bethel (1 Kings 12:26–29). Whether or not the god Yahweh was imagined as standing invisibly on the back of the golden calf as some have supposed, or if, which seems more likely, the Yahweh and Ba'al concepts had merged and Yahweh was depicted as a bull god is unimportant for our study. Hosea appears to be referring to some ritual in which the image of the god in animal form, whether it be Yahweh or Ba'al, was revered and kissed. On the other hand, if the mythic drama was acted out in the Ba'al shrines and there was a portrayal of the god's copulation with the animal, then Hosea may have been commenting on this situation.

Sexual acts with animals are more common in the Western world than most people know; but this behavior is not often discussed. Bestiality is more likely to occur on farms where there are an abundance of animals and opportunities for privacy that such sexual activity demands. Usually it is dogs, sheep, heifers, horses, pigs, and goats that are used sexually, but there are also reports of chickens, ducks, rabbits, and other small creatures being involved in such acts. Kinsey, in his sexuality studies, found that one-third of the educated males living in rural areas had sexual intercourse to the point of orgasm with animals.

R. E. L. Masters has published a number of personal narratives of men who have copulated with animals or who have subjected themselves to anal penetration by animals.[3] Some have brought animals to climax by masturbation and fellatio.

A somewhat newer phenomenon is that of sex between women and dogs in city settings. Woman-animal copulation is not new; only the situation is different. The dogs are pets that become sexual partners for lonely females, just as they have for males. Because of guilt and fear of social condemnation these activities are seldom discussed.

Masters indicates that in at least one instance the man experienced deep feelings of guilt because of the violation of biblical sexual taboos. He wrote to Masters and quoted from Hebrews 10:26–31. Subsequent correspondence indicated that he had overcome his guilt feelings and was continuing in his zoophilia.

All religious groups that use the Bible as a guide condemn bestiality. It is also against the law, and penalties vary from state to state and extend from fines to imprisonment. Despite the fact that some of those who admit to sexual involvement with animals suggest that the beasts were not unwilling partners, the human participant is held responsible. The beast is not killed, as in Mosaic law.

Folk tales abound about the birth to women or animals of offspring that combine human-animal features. There is absolutely no evidence that humans and animals can breed. R. E. L. Masters published a letter from a man who copulated with a pig. When a freak animal was born in the litter, the man believed it was his offspring. But deformed animals are not uncommon.

NOTES

1. *ANET*, p. 196 (laws 187, 188, 199, 200).
2. *ANET*, p. 139, col.i (v), Text I, AB.v.
3. R.E.L. Masters, *Sex-Driven People* (Los Angeles, 1966).
4. Ibid., pp. 121–210.

18

Prostitution

The Whore in Jewish Scriptures

An old maxim states that prostitution is the oldest profession in the world. Whether or not this is a statement of fact cannot be tested; but prostitution, the selling of sexual favors, is mentioned in the oldest literature from the ancient Near East, and references to it appear throughout the Bible.

The Hebrew term for prostitute or harlot or whore is *zonah*, which is derived from a root that suggests a person who is wanton, on the outside, and perhaps even repugnant. The whore was part of the community yet apart from it. She had human rights, but she was not fully respected. A priest could not marry a whore; she would render him unclean and unfit for service (Lev. 21:7, 14; 19:29). She was a blemished woman, and nothing blemished or imperfect could be associated with the worship of Yahweh (Lev. 22). She had been "pierced" by other men and was not a virgin. The money she was paid for her services could not be used to pay temple dues (Deut. 23:18). Should a priest's daughter become a whore, she was burned to death (Lev. 21:19). When the Hebrew writers condemned Israel for apostasy, they wrote of the nation "whoring" after other gods (Exod. 34:15; Lev. 17:7; 20:5; Num. 25:1; Judg. 2:17; etc.). The whore was not an honored woman.

We are not told how a woman became a whore. A law forbids a parent from making a whore out of his daughter: "Do not demean your daughter by making her a harlot" (Lev. 19:29). Just how this demeaning came about is not clear. Perhaps the daughter was sent out to earn money when the family became poor. Because the young woman was under the control of her father, there is a possibility that young women became whores at the behest of their fathers. It is also possible that orphaned girls or childless widows turned to prostitution for survival. The law protecting Hebrew maidens suggests that it was preferred that foreign women become whores.

When Tamar played the harlot and seduced Judah into intercourse, she wore a veil so she could not be recognized (Gen. 38:14). Because her situation was unique, it cannot be assumed that all harlots were veiled. Proverbs 7:10 makes reference to the "attire" of a prostitute, perhaps meaning the woman was veiled; but again this cannot be assumed as proven. Some scholars have suggested that the veiled whore signified her devotion to the fertility goddess Ishtar, but this is another speculation. In his angry denunciation of the nation's betrayal of Yahweh, Ezekiel said the nation exploited its beauty like a whore (Ezek. 16:10 ff.). Perhaps there was some distinctive garb for prostitutes, but there was also the tantalizing display of beauty and the promise of sexual adventure.

Business could be carried on in a tent at the side of the road as it was in the Tamar story. Jeremiah speaks of the nation as a harlot "sitting by the side of the road waiting to ensnare lovers" (Jer. 3:2). Apparently there were itinerant harlots. But there were also whorehouses. When the Hebrews sent spies into Jericho to assess the city's defenses, they spent most of the time in the home of Rahab the harlot (Josh. 2:1 ff.). When the city was destroyed, only Rahab and her family were spared (Josh. 6:17 ff.). Jeremiah referred to the men who frequented whorehouses (Jer. 5:7), and Ezekiel describes the whore with a couch on a raised platform, offering her body for the sexual satisfaction of any passerby. (Ezek. 16:25)

Some whores had children. A legend tells of two harlots who came to King Solomon for justice. They worked out of the same house and each had given birth to a child. During the night one infant was smothered to death when its mother rolled over on it. The complainant said that the first woman took the dead child and exchanged it for her living child. The first woman denied the charge and said the living child was hers. Solomon decided the case by offering to cut the child in two and give each mother one half. One woman agreed to take her half, the other begged that the child be spared and offered to give up her share. Solomon decided that the one who wanted the child to live was the real mother (1 Kings 3: 16–28). Many commentators have noted that he merely gave the child to the more compassionate woman, not necessarily the real mother. The point of the story, for this discussion, is that harlots also enjoyed civil rights.

The child of a harlot could become a leader. Jephthah was the son of a harlot, but he knew that his father was Gilead. He was prevented from having any claim to his father's estate, because his mother was a whore. Nevertheless, despite his parentage, he became a Hebrew hero (Judg. 11).

But harlots grow old, their beauty fades, and men forsake them. In an addition made to the writings of the prophet Isaiah, a writer included the song of the aged whore:

> Take a harp and wander about the city
> O forgotten whore.
> Produce sweet music and sing many songs
> So that you will be remembered

[Isa. 23:16]

The whore as a young woman would draw men to her by her beauty and their desire for her body, but now she can only attract attention by her music.

The Whore in Christian Scriptures

The word for "whore" in the Christian writings is the Greek term *porne*. Jesus referred to these women when he told a group of his countrymen in the temple that the hated tax-collector and the despised harlots would enter the kingdom of God before they did (Matt. 21:31). He was, of course, mocking their pious righteousness. In the parable of the prodigal son (Luke 15), Jesus had the older brother complain that the wayward son had spent his time, money, and energy on harlots (15:30). Jesus was aware of the presence of whores, of their business, and of the reality that they could relieve a young man of his money.

Prostitutes are not mentioned with approval in Christian writings. For Paul they are listed with immoral people, and to have intercourse with a whore is to be joined to the impure:

> Do you not know that your bodies are the organs of Christ? Shall I take then the organs of Christ and make them a whore's organ? Never! You know, do you not, that whoever joins himself to a whore becomes one body with her? For as it is written, "the two become one flesh." [1 Cor. 6:14 f.]

For Paul, sex with a whore rendered the person unclean.

The story of Rahab the harlot was used by Christian writers as a model of a person who was saved by faith and by works! The writer of Hebrews saw her as a model of faith:

> By faith, Rahab the harlot did not perish with those who disobeyed, because she gave a friendly welcome to the spies. [Heb. 11:31]

The writer of James suggested that Rahab's faith was not enough, that what really counted was what she did:

> And in the same way also, was not Rahab the harlot justified by works [deeds] when she received messengers and dispatched them by another way? For as the body apart from the spirit is dead, so faith without works [deeds] is dead. [James 2:25–26]

Cult Prostitutes

Sacred prostitution was part of the fertility religions of the ancient world. These religions sought to place humans in harmonious relationships with the life-generating forces of the cosmos, which had been personalized and given identities as gods and goddesses. The worship of these life-enhancing deities could be centered wherever the sacred or the holy was believed to have been manifested—by springs, at groves or trees, on the tops of hills and mountains. The purposes of the divine powers could be discerned in the flowing patterns of nature, from the flight of birds or the formation of clouds or in the internal organs of sacrificial animals.

Because the powers of nature had been personified as deities, the relational patterns between gods and goddesses were set forth in myths that were related to seasonal patterns. Winter would symbolize the death of the fertility deity; and spring, with the birth of new life, would represent the rebirth or resurrection of that same deity. The mating of animals in the flocks and herds would be enhanced by the mating of the fertility god and goddess in the mythic recitals.

Myths were dramatized in ritual; and what the gods did in the stories the cultic personae enacted in sacred drama. Because the gods copulated vigorously in joy of the body and the excitement of mating, so too the worshipers could become one with the harmonious flow of nature and enter into communion with the deified procreative powers by participating in sexual intercourse at the shrine with the servants of the deities who served as cult prostitutes.

The Hebrew terms used for these persons are derived from the root *q-d-s* which means "holy." The *qedeshim* (male cult prostitutes) and *qedeshoth* (female cult prostitutes) were sacred personnel, holy men and women who served their deities and their communities in shrines dedicated to strengthening the procreative powers of the cosmos for the benefit of humans.

The Hebrew concept of deity was far removed from this realm of thought. Yahweh was usually portrayed as a male deity without consorts. There are references that suggest that at times ideas about Yahweh melded with ideas about the Canaanite father-god Elyon or the fertility god Ba'al. For example, there is a reference to the "sons of God" (*bene ha elohim*) in Genesis 6:4. The same sort of reference is found in the Book of Job, where it is stated that the "sons of God" (*bene ha elohim*) presented themselves to their father-god Yahweh (Job 1:6, 2:1). In the creation myth in Genesis, there is reference to others besides God (*elohim*) being involved as consultants in the creation of humans (Gen. 1:26). Indeed, in one passage in Deuteronomy, Yahweh is portrayed as one of the sons of the most high god, the father-god Elyon:

> When Elyon gave the nations their inheritance
> When he separated humankind [the sons of Adam]
> He fixed the boundaries of the peoples [i.e., nations]
> According to the number of the sons of God
> Yahweh's share was his people,
> Jacob [i.e., Israel] his allotted inheritance.
>
> [Deut. 32:8]

These references contain fragments of ancient Hebrew mythic thought now lost to us, but they reflect that there was a time when, in certain Hebrew religious quarters, Yahweh was not always deemed to be a bachelor and was not always thought of as the supreme god. These mythic fragments do not represent the main thrust of Jewish scripture, which does at times portray Yahweh as one who manifests himself in storms and earthquakes (Judg. 5:4–5) but also as a deity in control of nature.

When the melding of concepts was at a peak, *qedeshim* and *qedeshoth* served in Yahweh's temple in Jerusalem and throughout the land; when purist monarchs were on the throne, there was a purging of the non-Yahweh elements (1 Kings 14:24; 15:12; 22:47; 2 Kings 23:7).

The nature of the fertility rituals is not clear, but the cult objects appear to have been a stone pillar (masculine) and a wooden pole or tree (feminine). Worshipers presented gifts to the shrine or the shrine deity, and before coinage was invented this could be in clothing, even clothing taken as a pledge for a debt (Amos 2:8); these very garments could be part of the bed on which the worship rites were performed. Wine was also given to the shrine, even wine taken as fines in the courts of the land; and like the clothing it became part of the worshipers' involvement in the cult as it was drunk in the holy place (Amos 2:8). The holy women at the shrine might be kept busy meeting the sexual and religious needs of the worshipers. Amos speaks of a man and his son going into the same woman (Amos 2:7). Hosea's wife, Gomer, became a devotee of the god Ba'al, and that prophet's preoccupation with the theme of adultery and harlotry reveals something of his personal anguish over Gomer's desertion.

Although there are no references to sacred prostitution in the Christian scriptures, it is known that the Mediterranean religions included sexual activities in their rites of worship, and Paul's insistence on sexual purity in the Christian converts is often set in contrast to what they had been (1 Cor. 6:9–11).

The Whore in Modern Society

Like her counterparts in the ancient world, the modern harlot is often a person who is a part of society and apart from it. She is recognized as "being there," and so long as her activities remain discreet she may not be troubled. When she and her companions take to the streets to solicit business in or near residential neighborhoods, she can quickly become a target for citizen protests and police action.

Most whores are victims. They come to their trade because of poverty. Young women come to large cities in pursuit of a career. They often find that the market is glutted with better-trained people; they are not needed or wanted, and their money dwindles. They move to poorer neighborhoods to economize on rent and find women like themselves engaging in prostitution to survive. They join the ranks.

But prostitution is a dangerous occupation. Psychopaths or men interested in "kinky" sex have inflicted grievous bodily harm on some of the women they have hired to entertain them for the evening. So pimps become the business managers of the whores, take most of the money earned in return for protection, room, board, and clothing, and perhaps give some semblance of caring for their "property." If the whore fails to bring in enough money ("turn enough tricks"), she may be beaten. Often drugs are involved, and once the young woman becomes "hooked" she is dependent upon her pimp as a drug supplier. She is then completely under his control.

Some women have become "madams," or managers of whorehouses. A madam's "girls" are looked after within the "house." Patrons are screened and the madam and her male bodyguards protect the young women from abuse by the patrons. Some madams are former prostitutes who, when they no longer felt attractive enough to draw customers, set themselves up in business as managers of younger whores.

There are different social levels within prostitution. The "streetwalker" is often considered to be the lowest level. She parades herself on public thoroughfares, hoping that someone will become interested in having sex with her. Above her are call-girls, who are contacted by regular customers or by carefully screened new customers by telephone. These women are often wined and dined before they are expected to spend the night with their host. Most are extremely beautiful and well educated, and some have regular jobs. There are also the "escort service" whores. Their advertisements appear in the yellow pages of the telephone directories in large cities, offering male and female "enthusiastic professionals for every occasion at your location for your convenience and plea-sure." Some offer massages. Most will accept payment by credit card. Whereas the streetwalker is often apprehended by the police, the call-girl and the escort services are much harder to prosecute.

As in the ancient world, there are both male and female prostitutes. They are available to either male or female customers. Males are handsome young men with good physiques. They are expected to be sexually vigorous and willing and able to accommodate most of the demands of their male or female clients.

None of these are welcomed by society in general or by religious organiza-tions. Some people suggest that prostitutes perform a service in providing a way for men and women to relieve their sexual tensions and satisfy their sexual desires without violence or rape. The streetwalkers do present some unique social prob-lems in neighborhoods where other women may be accosted by men looking for whores. The women become upset, the husbands and fathers become angry, and the citizenry takes action. For Jews and Christians, prostitutes are sinners. They have forsaken the way of the Bible and the mores of the society and have become repugnant figures who do not deserve respect. On the other hand, there are within religious organizations and certainly within humanist groups those who recognize these women and men as victims of society. Most whores say that they are in the business to earn a living. Some few will say they enjoy the work; most say they do not. Many are hooked on drugs and need the money to support their habit. Some of the young men are in debt or in trouble with the law and need money to repay borrowed funds or to hire an attorney. Some of the women are saving money in the hope that the time will come when they will be able to settle down in a respectable home—perhaps with children they have borne.

Their patrons are often lonely, isolated individuals who seek companionship for a short time, who feel the need to be touched, and who use the sexual outlet as a momentary expression of affection for a partner they have never seen before and probably will not see again. There is a pathological dimension in the present setting that reflects on the social conditions that promote this way of life and the personal isolation that causes individuals to turn to whores for human contact.

Sometimes there are devoted members of the clergy as well as lay people who develop a mission to help the whores. They work among them, seeking to help them break with their profession and find suitable employment. Many seek to convert the whores to a particular belief system, many others simply try to help. They find their motivation in biblical teachings about compassion.

19

Illegitimacy

The term *bastard* refers to a child born to unwed parents and who can therefore be considered to be the product of an illegal or illegitimate union. A bastard is an "illegitimate child." The oft-quoted maxim that there are in reality no illegitimate children but only illegitimate parents contains a basic truth, but that truth does not operate in our society. It is the child who bears the label of "bastard." It is the child who is considered "illegitimate." It is the child and often the child's mother who must bear the condemnation of family, society, and religion, although the father may bear some social embarrassment.

An example of public reaction to children born out of wedlock occurred in 1982 when California State Senator John G. Schmitz admitted publicly that he had fathered two children out of wedlock. The newspaper headlines read in large bold type: "Schmitz has two Illegitimate Children."[1] The children, not the parents, were labeled. Indeed, one of Schmitz's conservative colleagues, Representative E. Dannemeyer, almost justified the senator's behavior. He allegedly told a *Los Angeles Times* reporter that "at least it shows a preference by him for heterosexual life style." The report goes on to say that Dannemeyer "then talked angrily against homosexuals and their political activism, contending that the acceptance of that activism is 'a story and an issue more profound' than the revelations about Schmitz."[2] By diverting the issue, Dannemeyer came close to exonerating Schmitz and left the burden of the label of illegitimacy untouched, to be carried by the mother and the two children. There is little doubt that the effect of the disclosure will affect Schmitz's political career and perhaps also his family life, but time will tend to obscure the extramarital affair; the two children, the victims, will be labeled for life.

The Bible also labeled the child and condemned the child's descendants. The Deuteronomic law stated:

> A bastard [*mamzer*] shall not enter Yahweh's congregation, even to the tenth generation he shall not enter Yahweh's congregation. [Deut. 23:2]

118

The term *mamzer* refers to children born out of any union not approved by Jewish law, including those born out of wedlock or of incestuous marriage, and so on. The term could be expanded. Although the word *mamzer* is not used, it is possible that the warrior hero Jephthah, whose mother was a whore, could have been considered to be a bastard. He was driven from his home by the legitimate sons of his father, who told him: "You have no inheritance in our father's home; you are another woman's son" (Judg. 11:2).

Bastard could be used as a deprecating label. The word *mamzer* is used in Zechariah 9:6 to describe the people who would settle the Philistine town of Ashod. The Christian writer of Hebrews believed that the true sons of God would be recognized by their willingness to face discipline; bastards (*nothoi*) would be those who failed in the test of sonship.

There is some slight evidence in the Gospels that there was a cloud over Jesus' birth. The idea of supernatural impregnation by the Holy Spirit might have been acceptable on a mythological level, but not biologically when one was confronted with a contemporary human being. The Gospel of Matthew states that Joseph was preparing to divorce Mary, Jesus' mother, to whom he was betrothed but with whom he had not consummated the marriage. But he had a dream in which an angelic figure informed him that Mary was pregnant by the Holy Spirit (Matt. 1:18–25). The implication is that Joseph suspected that she had been involved with another man and that the child within her was not his and would therefore be a bastard—an illegitimate child.

In the Gospel of John, the Pharisees are said to have asked Jesus, "Where is your father?" (John 8:19), and perhaps there is an implied question about Jesus' paternity. However, it is possible that those who have called attention to this verse place too much emphasis on its historicity. It is easier to understand the statement as part of the theological proclamation by the gospel writer in which he creates situations and statements rather than reports them. This gospel is generally dated near the end of the first century C.E. and was not written by anyone who knew or heard Jesus personally.

Because Christian theology placed emphasis upon the miraculous impregnation of Mary, little attention was given to Jesus' paternity. It was assumed, despite the fact that the idea of divine impregnation of earthly women was a fairly common literary device, that in Jesus' case the Holy Spirit was the male parent. Liberal scholars generally assume that Jesus was the son of Joseph and that only as the theology of the church developed did the idea of a divine birth and the "Son of God" mythology come into being. If the statement in Matthew has any basis in fact, it is possible that Jesus was an illegitimate child, a Jewish *mamzer*.

One can only imagine what might have happened throughout the past centuries if the Christian church had kept this issue open and had acknowledged that its founder, Jesus, may have been a bastard. No doubt children who were labeled "bastard" because of what their parents had done or had not done in failing to be married would have been accepted as full human beings, and perhaps relieved of a damaging label. The insistence upon the supernatural obscured the natural, and children born out of wedlock were deprived of a hero figure who might have helped to raise their social status and relieve them of the stigma.

Although the term *mamzer* can be applied directly to children born of unmarried parents, it can be extended to include any marriage that falls outside of Orthodox Jewish ecclesiastical definitions. For example, in 1972 in Israel, Rabbi Schlomo Goren, chief rabbi for Ashkenazi (Western) Jews, approved the marriages of an Israeli brother and sister who had been considered *mamzerim* (bastards or outcasts) because their mother had not been divorced from her first husband in the manner prescribed by Jewish law.[3] The children were labeled because of what the mother had failed to do.

The term *bastard* has had a varied history in Western culture. At times it was considered to be a serious reflection on the nature of the person so labeled. A family was not allowed to forget it if a grandparent or a great uncle had been born to parents who were not married, and that whole branch of the family was tainted with this heritage. It was as though the Deuteronomic code had become part of the culture and there was intent to fulfill the ruling that the sins of the father would be upon the children to the third and fourth generation (Deut. 5:9) and mark the descendants of the bastard to the tenth generation.

Hostility to illegitimacy reflects reaction against behavior that is seen to be a threat against the legitimate family system. It is labeled "immoral" because it challenges accepted mores. It has been condemned by most conservative religious groups and, because such organizations tend to be followers rather than leaders in social change—preferring to support the status quo as a divine given—attention is given to fulfillment of divinely revealed rules rather than to human need.

Most societal criticism is directed against the child and the unwed mother. The mother and child are sociological phenomena; the father is not. Because the mother carries the child in her womb for nine months and her pregnant state announces that she was engaged in sexual relationships outside of marriage, she is open to attack. The responsibilities of raising the child most often fall upon the unwed mother and, because she may require welfare to survive, she is again an object for attack. Should she seek male companionship to help alleviate her loneliness, she may again become pregnant by her new lover and engender further criticism.

It has been stated often that attacks on welfare mothers and unwed mothers and their children are thinly disguised expressions of racial prejudice. The social system that forces minorities into perpetual poverty through low-paying jobs that have no security also produces disproportionate rates of illegitimacy. Because blacks are the largest ethnic minority, unwed black women and their children often become the focus of social criticism.

The criticism may also reflect the uneasiness of middle-class families as they feel the problem of illegitimacy come closer to their own lives. Most of these families can afford abortions and are willing to have their daughters undergo abortions should they become pregnant, even when religious beliefs are opposed to abortion. The social embarrassment is too much to contemplate. One wealthy Roman Catholic family sent their daughter to visit abroad and have her baby there after the teen-aged girl became pregnant. The baby was then turned over to an adoption agency. The guilt over bearing a child out of wedlock and of releasing her baby for adoption, the awareness of the family embarrassment and feelings of shame over her sexual involvement, and the guilt stemming from her Catholic upbringing and her feelings of having compromised her faith produced deep trauma for which the young woman required extensive therapy.

A seventeen-year-old Mormon girl, pregnant out of wedlock, planned to violate her church's teaching and have an abortion. She sought counsel from her bishop, who promptly blessed the unborn child in her womb. She was in deep conflict. How could she abort a fetus that had received the blessing of the church? At the same time, how could she continue her education, move among her Mormon companions and live comfortably in her Mormon family with her pregnancy?

Not every family can gracefully accept a daughter who has born a child out of wedlock, and not every family is able to make a child feel welcome at all levels at all times. Ghosts in family closets creep out in shadowy references to haunt lives. The shame felt by some families and the belief that the daughter has sinned together with the biblical injunctions about bastards meld to form tenaciously held attitudes that can be expressed in subtle ways in family circles. It is seldom that an illegitimate father has comparable pressures.

In recent years new facets have been added to the issue of illegitimacy. Many couples now live together and raise families while ignoring the legal contracts and licensing associated with formal marriage. The man and the woman love one another and care for their families. They believe that the quality of the relationship constitutes a true marriage. Problems may arise concerning the status of the children. For example, in some court cases involving the deaths of "illegitimate" children damages have been denied to the parents that would ordinarily have been awarded had they been married. "Illegitimate" children have also been denied damages in a case involving negligence in the death of their mother. If the father dies without leaving a will, inheritance problems can develop and his "family" may be denied their claims despite the fact that he had lived with, supported, and cared for these "illegitimate" offspring and his "unmarried" wife. Even in the Social Security system, which provides for children born out of wedlock, there may be discrimination.

In Sweden, labels like "illegitimate" and "bastard" and the prejudices associated with them have been abandoned, but in most Western countries the stigma remains. Unwed mothers and their children experience unique social and economic pressures, such as the hostility of hospital clerks who fill out birth certificates, difficulty in getting insurance coverage or help from public services, and problems in finding employment.

The father may also face problems. Should an unwed mother decide to give up her child for adoption and should the child's natural father wish to adopt the infant, he may discover he has no legal rights to the child. When parents are not married, the mother and the child form the social unit recognized as "the family."

A number of women who are prominent public personalities as well as some who are not well known have announced that they will bear children out of wedlock. Recently a forty-year-old psychologist became pregnant by sperm obtained from the California based "Nobel Prize" sperm bank. The operators of the "bank" assumed that she was married. She was not, and she publicly declared her joy in the experience of bearing a child.

The attitudes of most conservative religious leaders reflect anything but enthusiasm for pregnant unmarried women. One cannot know to what extent the Deuteronomic attitude toward bastards remains the inheritance of religion in our present society. While Mother Theresa worked in India, responding to human need among the poor and the outcast, the legitimate and the illegitimate, without discrimination, the religious hierarchy blessed her work. But it failed to make any statements that would help to change attitudes toward children who, in an enlightened society, can still be called "bastards" because their parents failed to conform to accepted marriage customs.

There are those who believe that the policy of the Roman Catholic church on the annulment of marriages produces more "bastards" than out-of-wedlock births. Roman Catholics who have been married by a priest and who later go through a civil divorce to dissolve the marriage cannot be remarried to other persons by the church unless the first marriage is annulled by the church. In other words, according to canon law, the church can pronounce certain marriages null and void, implying that for one reason or another the marriage is believed to have never been properly consummated. In the minds of many Roman Catholics, this nullification implies that the marriage never really existed. What happens to the status of children born to a couple whose marriage has been nullified? If their parents were never "properly married" are these children "bastards"? In the eyes of many, they are, and the stigma is a troubling one. Moreover, with the failure of marriages approaching one out of two, the basis for annulment has been broadened to the extent that in most cases no real problem exists for those seeking official church recognition of the divorce. Clearly, until the Roman Catholic church publicly clarifies its position concerning the legitimacy of marriages that are later annulled and recognizes the legitimacy of divorce (rather than annulment), the question of the legitimacy of the children will continue to be a troublesome issue.

NOTES

1. *Los Angeles Times*, July 21, 1982.
2. *Los Angeles Times*, July 22, 1982.
3. According to an Associated Press report in the *Los Angeles Times*, November 21, 1972.

20

Abortion

References to natural abortion or miscarriage do appear in the Bible, but there is no mention of the evacuation of the womb by unnatural means apart from the curse placed on a woman accused of adultery (see chapter 14). One Hebrew law deals with a miscarriage due to injury:

> When men fight with one another and injure a pregnant woman causing a miscarriage, and no further harm follows, the one who injured her shall be fined according to what the husband demands of him . . . . [Exod. 21:22].

The condition of the woman is noted, and it can be assumed that, should she die or be crippled, an additional fine or perhaps a charge of manslaughter would be invoked. The payment is not to the woman as the injured person, but to the husband to whom she belongs for his loss of a child. On the scale of valuation of males and females set forth in Leviticus 27:1–8, the fine the husband might demand would vary according to whether the aborted fetus was male or female.

There are several biblical references to "untimely births" that may mean miscarriages. Job, in his misery, laments that he was not stillborn (3:11); then he asks:

> Why was I not hidden like an untimely birth like an infant that never sees light. (3:16)

The reference to hiding the untimely birth appears to refer to the disposal of the fetus. A Psalmist cursing the wicked calls upon Yahweh to cause them to disappear like an "untimely birth" (58:8), which again suggests the secret or private disposal of a fetus. The writer of Ecclesiastes claims that if a person does not get satisfaction out of life and doesn't even get a decent burial he is worse off than the "untimely birth" (Eccles. 6:3).

In the modern controversy over abortion neither side can draw directly upon biblical verses to support its position. Those who oppose abortion often quote the commandment "Thou shalt not kill," which has given rise to a debate about when the fetus can be said to be a living person with a separate identity that could be "killed." The story of the creation of Adam in Genesis states that he was a clay figurine until Yahweh blew into his nostrils the "breath of life," causing him to become a "living being" (2:7). This would suggest that until a fetus is able to sustain life independent of the mother, it lacks personhood.

On the other hand, those who would argue that the fetus is a person and is entitled to full protection under the law state that at the very moment that the sperm penetrates the ovum the soul enters the fertilized egg and that it is the soul that gives personal identity. Of course the soul is an intangible mythic entity, an article of faith for whose existence there is absolutely no evidence. If one believes in the existence of the soul, then it is possible to argue that the soul enters the fertilized egg or that the soul does not become a part of the person until the infant emerges from the womb and breathes on its own.

The Hebrews thought of themselves as psychosomatic units—they did not distinguish between body and soul in the sense that a person had a soul; they saw the person as an animated body, a breathing, alive body. The person was a unit, a body-soul. It was in the developing Christian church that the idea of the separate identities of body and soul was developed. On the basis of biblical literature it is impossible to support the idea of the soul entering the body at any specific time. Nor is it possible to argue that the fetus is a "person" on the basis of biblical teachings. The debate about abortion is centered in theological opinion and belief.

21

Exhibitionism

The tenth-century B.C.E. Hebrew creation-myth tells of Adam and Eve in the Garden of Eden and notes that "they were both naked and were not ashamed" (Gen. 2:25). In this primal state of existence, they were like the other created creatures, like the animals and birds, with only their own skin as covering. But, when Eve ate of the forbidden fruit of the tree of knowledge of good and evil, humans were no longer in the state of animal innocence—they now knew what divine beings knew—and they discovered they were naked. Eve was the enlightener, and from that time on, according to the myth, humans had to cover their genitals—first with fig leaves, then with animal skins presented by Yahweh and taken from the animals, from whom the couple were now estranged. The naked body had become a taboo.

Some biblical passages that refer to the exposure of the human body imply engagement in a sexual act. To uncover another's nakedness meant to engage in intercourse and not merely to look at a naked body. The uncovering of another's nakedness can also mean to humiliate that person and to shame and demean the individual. The expression is often used when a writer wishes to threaten the nation (Israel or Judah) depicted as the bride or wife of the deity. In anger, Yahweh would expose the woman's genitals to make her the laughing stock of other nations. Although there is no reference to what is currently called "indecent exposure," the biblical taboo against uncovering another's nakedness or viewing another's nakedness, as well as the emphasis on the necessity to cover the genitals, exerts a conditioning effect on present-day Christians and Jews.

When King David sent emissaries to the Ammonite kingdom, King Hannum and his court advisors suspected that David's men were really military spies whose purpose was to determine the strengths and weaknesses of the capital city as part of the preparation for an attack. The envoys were sent back to Jerusalem in disgrace. Half of the beard was shaved from each man's face and his garments were sheared off at the waist, exposing the genitals. This humiliating exposure triggered a war (2 Sam. 10).

King David was responsible for bringing the sacred ark to the city of Jerusalem, thereby converting a political capital into a religious center for the worship of Yahweh. The entry rites included sacrifices and ecstatic dancing. David, clothed only in an ephod—a short linen apron that covered only the forepart of his body but not the back—danced ''with all his might'' so that his genitals were exposed. His first wife, Michal, the daughter of King Saul, watched from a palace window and was disgusted. When David returned to the palace, flushed with excitement, she scornfully commented:

> How the King of Israel did honor to himself today, exposing himself before his servants' women as some uncouth boor exposes himself. [2 Sam. 6:20]

David's angry response mocked the failure of Michal's family to retain the throne and threatened even more socially humiliating acts in the future. Michal appears to have been separated from the king from that moment on, for the text notes that she never bore a child (2 Sam. 6:23).

David's dance was part of a ritual—a cultic ritual associated with the ark of the covenant. The text notes that he leapt and whirled in his performance. If, as some scholars have argued, the bringing of the ark into Jerusalem was ritualized and dramatized each year, it is quite possible that sacred dancing was part of the reenactment, but genital exposure may have been eliminated from subsequent observances.

Another account tells of total exposure of the body by King Saul in a ritual associated with Yahwism (1 Sam. 19:18–24). Saul had been pursuing David and learned that the future king was at Naioth. He sent soldiers to seize David, but they came under the influence of a company of prophets led by the great seer Samuel and failed to carry out their mission. A second and third band also came under the influence of Samuel and ''prophesied.'' Saul himself came and fell under the prophetic spell. In ecstatic frenzy he stripped his clothes from his body and lay naked for a day and a night.

Saul was responsive to rapture-producing influences in another account. Having been secretly anointed for kingship by the prophet Samuel, he encountered a band of prophets (1 Sam. 10:1–13). This group used harps, tambourines, flute, and lyres to produce frenzied responses. How much of the transformation of personality can be traced to Canaanite religion and how much was indigenous Yahwism cannot be determined at this time.

Priests who served at the altar of Yahweh had to have their genitals covered. They were required to wear linen pants (Exod. 20:26, 28:42). The reasons for the genitals' having to be covered when the priest approached the altar are not known. If the outer priestly garment covered the body from the shoulders down, why was an inner garment needed? Could the divinity associated with the holy altar be offended by what could be viewed from below? No one seems to know the answer, but clearly there is a reenforcement of the taboo against exposure of genitalia.

Full naked exposure could be used to dramatize the dangers of alliances between Judah and foreign nations in acts that today would be labeled ''public protest.'' In the last part of the eighth century B.C.E., a number of small states formed an alliance to withstand the pressure of paying taxes to the mighty nation of Assyria. King Hezekiah of Judah was eager to join the rebels, but the prophet Isaiah believed destruction by Assyria would result. He paraded naked through the streets of Jerusalem to demonstrate what would be the fate of anyone who resisted Assyria (Isaiah 20). There was no condemnation of his act and he appears to have violated no taboo, because prophets, believed to be acting according to the divine will, seem to have been placed in a special category and their socially abnormal acts were in keeping with their calling.

Warnings of punishment often contained the threat of exposure of private parts. Isaiah warned the women of Jerusalem who appeared to be indifferent to the military threats to the city that their god Yahweh would ''lay bare their private parts'' (Isa. 5:17). Because Hosea and subsequent prophets portrayed the nations of Israel and Judah as wives or brides of Yahweh who had betrayed their marriage vows, threats of punishment by being overcome by foreign nations often refer to the exposure of female genitals (Hos. 2:3, 10). The imagery could be applied to other nations. Isaiah (47:3) threatened Babylon with exposure, and Nahum (3:5) mocked the Assyrians when Nineveh was destroyed by the Medes and Babylonians and promised that the city's genitals would be displayed.

One curious episode involving nudity is recorded in the Gospel of Mark. When Jesus was arrested, an unidentified young man wearing only a linen cloth about his body was also seized by the mob. He fled naked, leaving his covering in the hands of his would-be captors (Mark 14:51). Scholars have puzzled over the identity of the man, and the reason why the story was included, without arriving at satisfactory answers. No negative interpretation seems to be given to the nakedness of the young man.

Indecent Exposure and Exhibitionism

In our modern society, television shows have made the exhibitionist or ''flasher'' a comedy figure. The individual is usually portrayed as an aging male, wearing a long raincoat. It is assumed that the audience understands that the man is naked beneath the coat. At the proper moment in the comedy the man pulls back the coat and presumably exposes his genitals to some horrified female. The audience laughs.

What is obscured by this kind of presentation is the fear and shock experienced by many women and by many children who have experienced this kind of behavior. Moreover, the implication that the ''flasher'' is always an aging male reinforces the unfortunate image of the ''dirty old man'' who is both lascivious and rather sick. It is true that some of those convicted of indecent exposure have been aging males; it is also true that many have been young or middle-aged.

Indecent exposure refers to the ''unlawful exposure of 'private parts' to public view.''[1] In the privacy of one's home an individual is free to parade in the nude, provided the shades are drawn and no one from the outside is able to watch. But even here the legal ramifications are not clear. If a male walks naked about the house and a woman sees him from the street and reports him, he may be charged with indecent exposure. If a woman walks about her home in the nude and is seen from the street by a male, he may be accused of being a ''peeping Tom.'' The assumption is that the man is parading himself with lascivious intent, while the woman is an innocent victim. Perhaps there is some basis in fact for this prejudgment. Most reported cases of indecent exposure involve males who expose their genitals in public places to women or children.

The location and mode of exhibiting the genitals varies. Sometimes it happens in alleys, sometimes on public thoroughfares. Sometimes a man stops his car and asks a woman or girl standing on the curb for directions and, when she approaches the car to respond, she discovers that he is naked from the waist down or has opened the front of his pants and is masturbating or fondling himself. His intention is to be seen. Although about one-third of reported sex offenses are cases of indecent exposure, it is believed that many more incidents go unreported. Individuals who have been arrested often confess that they have exposed themselves many times before and give times and places that can be checked against police records of complaints. Because some of these confessions tally with complaints, it is possible that some of those that cannot be checked have some basis in fact. Some women will not bother to report an incident because they are too embarrassed to talk about it to the police or because they believe it is something that is not very serious. Young children are sometimes too embarrassed to talk about it, but when they do the parents often file reports to protect their child and other children.

Exactly what prompts a man to expose himself is not clear. Some appear to get some sort of sexual satisfaction from the very act of exhibiting their genitals. Some masturbate after the act. Some hope that a woman will be excited and will respond sexually, just as they would should she expose herself.

NOTE

1. John M. Macdonald, *Indecent Exposure* (Springfield, 1973), p. 3.

22

Homosexuality

Homosexuality, which became known as "the sin that dares not speak its name," seems to be as old as human history. The term *homosexual* appears to have been coined in 1869 by Karl Maria Benkert (Karoly M. Kertbeny), an Austrian homosexual-rights advocate, in a pamphlet attacking the Prussian sodomy law. The word *gay* is older and is derived from the Old Provencal *gai*. By the nineteenth century, the English counterpart "gay" had acquired a slang meaning that implied "immoral," and when applied to women signified "prostitute."[1]

The attitude of the Christian church toward homosexuality has fluctuated greatly throughout the past 1,900 years. During the Middle Ages, some clergy wrote erotic poetry expressing the sexual feelings of one male for another. At the other extreme were scholars like Thomas Aquinas who could envision homosexual acts as "vices against nature" and "unnatural." In recent times, with the emergence of homosexuals from "the closet," the status of homosexuals has assumed new importance. There are those who would deny homosexuals their full rights as citizens and persons, and there are religious organizations that would bar homosexuals from membership and from holding any office within the church structure.

Homosexuality is viewed differently by different groups. Some would label it a personality disorder, some a perversion, some a sin. The *Psychiatric Dictionary* defines it as "the state of being in love with one belonging to the same sex" and also, separating female and male aspects, as "erotic or genital relationship between two (or more) males."[2] Homosexuals use different language in defining themselves. Don Clark, in *Loving Someone Gay*, writes:

> I am Gay and that means that I know I am able to involve myself emotionally, sensuously, erotically and intellectually with someone of the same gender. He and I can interrelate in a whole and satisfying way without having to create dishonesty and diversion from fear of possible sexuality. Being Gay means that I know I am *capable* of this range of relating to another male and that I am *willing* to act on the capability and translate this potential into behavior. [Italics in original.][3]

Some would include bisexuals under the label of homosexuality. Bisexuals are those can enjoy sexual intimacy with either male or female partners.

Homosexuality in the Bible

Biblical writers portray homosexuality as offensive to both societal and religious mores. Sexual relationships between males may have been tolerated in the towns of Gibeah, Sodom, and Gomorrah, and perhaps homosexuality was common in Canaanite communities; but the biblical references to these places and patterns serve as warnings to Jews and Christians that homosexuality is unacceptable behavior.

One Noah legend states that Ham, Noah's son, took advantage of his father when Noah was drunk (Gen. 9:18–27). The actual text states only that Ham "saw his father's nakedness," referring to the sexual organs. It is possible that only viewing the genitals is meant, or perhaps he had sexual relations with him. The text goes on to say that, when Noah awoke and discovered what his son "had done to him," he cursed Ham and condemned his descendants to servitude. It might seem that this curse was something of an overreaction to Ham's almost accidental viewing of his parent's genitals! The reference to what Ham "had done to him" may imply something more than casual looking.

Of course the legend is etiological; it explains why certain relationships came about. Shem is the eponymous ancestor of the Semites and the Hebrew people (Gen. 10:21; 11:10–31). Ham is the ancestor of Canaan. The Hebrews were conquerors of the Canaanites. Because this story was incorporated into the temple literature during the time of Solomon, it indicates that the conquest of Canaan was not simply happenstance, nor the result of Hebrew military superiority; the conquest was fulfillment of an ancient curse that an angry father (Noah) had placed on his son (Ham) and the son's descendants (Canaan).

Sodom and Gomorrah

The story of the destruction of Sodom and Gomorrah (Gen. 19) is one in a collection of sagas associated with the patriarch Abraham. Again the legend is etiological: it explains the destruction of these cities of the plain as a supernatural act. Although it is still debatable, it is quite possible that the city of Sodom is mentioned in the third-millennium texts discovered by Italian excavators at ancient Ebla in Syria. Biblical references are so obscure that debates will continue among scholars as to the exact location of these ancient sites. Because they appear to be located in the southern region of the Dead Sea, it is possible that ignition of seepage of natural gas, oil, and bitumin, which are found in the great rift valley of the Dead Sea, caused the destruction of the towns. The biblical account of the event registers a moral judgment on the non-Hebrew inhabitants of the cities and claims they were destroyed by the Hebrew god, Yahweh.

The legend records the visit of two angels to the Canaanite city of Sodom to investigate outcries against the violence in the city. Lot, Abraham's nephew, provided hospitality, which in ancient Near East tradition signified that the visitors were under his protection. The males of the city of Sodom surrounded Lot's house and demanded that the guests be delivered to them to be used sexually. Lot offered his two virgin daughters as substitutes. The angelic visitors rescued themselves and the young women by using supernatural power to cause the Sodomites to become temporarily blind. Subsequently, Yahweh destroyed Sodom and the neighboring city of Gomorrah by "fire and brimstone."

Gibeah

A similar story with quite different consequences was told about the Hebrew town of Gibeah (Judg. 19). In this instance, a Levite and his concubine were provided shelter by an old man. As in the Sodom account, the males of Gibeah demanded the Levite for their sexual pleasure. No supernatural powers were available in this story, and the Levite pushed his concubine out of the door to satisfy the lust of the men of Gibeah. They abused her until she died. The result of this violent action was civil war and the ultimate destruction of the city.

Clearly there are similarities in the two stories. Both deal with violence and the attempted rape of transient males by villagers. In one instance the aggressors are Canaanites; in the other they are Hebrews. In the Gibeah narrative, the lustful violence ended with the death of a woman; in the other, supernatural magic provided protection.

Male and female rape are symbols of the dissolution of, or the absence of, respect for another's personhood. When such behavior becomes local custom, it reflects communal sociopathology that uses community power to violate an individual sexually. There is nothing in either story to suggest that the mores of either town prohibited homosexuality or, indeed, mass rape. Because the accounts state that all the townsmen were involved, one might conclude that both homosexuality and the rape of outsiders were approved behavior.

It is possible to argue that the Hebrews of Gibeah adopted the ways of Canaan as reflected in the stories of Noah (Ham symbolized Canaan) and Sodom. In any case, rape, the violent sexual use of an individual by a mob, the disregarding of the protection that the town should have given to guests who were taken under the roof of one of the inhabitants, and murder by rape were simply not to be tolerated. The behavior of the men of Gibeah was condemned and punished by the larger community; Sodom, according to the Hebrew legend, was destroyed by divine action.

Cult Prostitution

Male cult-prostitutes participated in worship rites in some shrines in ancient Israel, and the implication is that shrines were dedicated to the worship of Yahweh, the Hebrew God. The strong denunciations of these persons by Israelite purists, who considered their role abominable and not part of traditional Hebrew worship, makes it clear that the idea of male prostitution came from the outside, from the practices in Canaan.

The term translated "male cult-prostitute" is the Hebrew word *qadesh*, which simply indicates that they were "holy" men engaged in work associated with the sacred (cf. 1 Kings 14:24). From time to time efforts were made to purge foreign elements, including cult prostitution, from temple rites. Both King Asa (1 Kings 15:12) and King Jehoshaphat (1 Kings 22:46) are mentioned with approval because they abolished cult prostitution, but subsequent monarchs (who did not receive editorial approval) reinstituted the custom. The patterns of purging and re-institution apparently continued right up to the time of King Josiah (638–609 B.C.E.), after which the Solomonic temple was destroyed (2 Kings 23:7).

The Deuteronomic law, the law that most scholars believe was composed during the seventh century, came to light during the refurbishing of the temple, when King Josiah began to remove the foreign elements. The code stated

> There shall be no female cult prostitute [*qedeshah*] from the daughters of Israel and no male cult prostitute [*qadesh*] from the sons of Israel. You shall not bring the earnings of a whore [*zonah*], nor the wages of a dog [*keleb*] into the house of Yahweh your god. [Deut. 23:17–18]

It is clear that the Deuteronomic writer is paralleling *qedeshah* (female cult-prostitute) and *zonah* (common whore) and *qadesh* (male cult prostitute) with *keleb* (dog).[4] Thus *qadesh* and *keleb* may be interchangeable terms, and male cult-prostitutes were labeled "dogs" by Hebrew worshipers of Yahweh.[5]

The exact role of the male cult-prostitute is never made clear. There can be little doubt that the Hebrews borrowed the concept of cult prostitution from the Canaanites. Canaanite religion was centered in fertility and reproduction. The *qedeshim* belonged to the temple cult and participated in rites designed to stimulate divine help in increasing fertility in the soil and in the flocks and herds.[6] Whether or not homosexual acts were involved cannot be known for sure. It is possible that the *qedeshim* were castrated sodomites (cf. Deut. 23:2). What is clear is that there existed in ancient Israel a diversity of beliefs and practices concerning cultic rites and social mores. The Bible preserves the point of view of those opposed to cult prostitution and homosexuality.

Opposition to homosexuality is expressed legalistically in Leviticus 18:22:

> Thou shalt not lie with [have sexual intercourse with] a male as with a woman, it is an abomination.

The death penalty is invoked as punishment for such an act in Leviticus 20:13:

> If a man lies with [has sexual intercourse with] a male as with a woman, they have both committed an abomination and must be killed, their blood is on them.

Because these rulings appear in the context of laws forbidding participation in non-Jewish practices, it is possible to suggest that one aim of the laws is to protect Jews from drifting into association with the religious practices associated with other gods.

Inasmuch as these laws are said to have been given by Yahweh to Moses, they bear the stamp of "revealed truth." Divine reprisal is threatened if the regulations are violated (Lev. 26:3–45).

Homosexuality in Christian Scriptures

In a letter written to the Christian community in Corinth about the middle of the first century of the common era, the apostle Paul wrote:

> Don't be misled, neither the immoral nor idolators nor adulterers nor effeminate men nor sodomites [*malakoi oute arsenokoitai*] nor thieves nor drunkards nor robbers will inherit God's Kingdom. [1 Cor. 6:9]

Paul uses two terms for homosexual partners, indicating the one who submits and the one who performs.[7]

In his letter to the Christian community in Rome, in a polemic against what he deemed to be idolatry, Paul condemned homosexuality. He believed like the writers of Jewish scripture, that worship of non-Jewish gods led to moral corruption. As a consequence of this idolatry, he claimed:

> God abandoned them to their degrading passions. Their women exchanged natural relations for unnatural and the men too in the same way gave up natural relations with women and were consumed with passion for one another, men committing shameless acts with men and receiving in their own person the inevitable penalty for their perversity. [Rom. 1:27]

Both homosexuality and lesbianism are condemned as immoral in this statement. Exactly what Paul meant by the "penalty" is not clear—perhaps some form of infection or venereal disease.

Both the Corinthian letter and the Roman letter were written to newly formed Christian groups that included new converts with varied backgrounds. Paul believed that, when one joined the Christian movement, the past was abandoned and former beliefs, customs, and behavior patterns unacceptable to the Jewish-Christian mores as expressed in Jewish scripture were no longer accepted or practiced. The Corinthian converts had at one time been involved in one or more of the activities he condemned. He wrote to the Corinthians and the Romans as a teacher to instruct in matters of faith. His letters confronted issues that were specific problems in these new churches. Later, when his letters were gathered and became part of the authoritative scripture of the Christian movement, they were given authority and assumed a universality that went far beyond their original localized settings. They now applied to Christians everywhere. Paul's attitude to homosexuality, which seems to have been the attitude of other leaders in the Christian church, became the official position of Christianity.

The writer of the letter called I Timothy listed homosexuals (*arsenokoitais*) among the godless and irreligious together with murderers (1:10). If, as many New Testament scholars believe, the writing is post-Pauline, it is clear that the attitudes expressed in Paul's correspondence with Corinth and Rome were still those of the expanding church. This letter, one of a group known as "pastorals," was directed to leaders of the developing Christian communities and contributed to the continued opposition of the early Christians to homosexuality.

The little tract called Jude, which was probably composed near the end of the first century, is an exhortation and polemic "for the faith once delivered to the saints" and is opposed to those who, among other things, "defile the flesh." Like other early Christian writers, the author used Jewish scriptures as a source for examples of doom that would overtake sinners, and he does not hesitate to interpret his sources in the light of his Christian beliefs. In verse 7, Sodom and Gomorrah are mentioned as examples of unnatural lust:

> . . . just as Sodom and Gomorrah and the neighboring cities which acted likewise
> indulged in immorality and went after strange flesh [homosexuality] serve as an
> example by undergoing a punishment of eternal fire.

The writer has added a new feature to the story—eternal damnation. The idea of punishment in the afterlife was not part of the early Hebrew belief-system and was incorporated into some sects of Judaism in the few centuries preceding the beginnings of Christianity. It became a central part of Christian belief. The author of the Book of Jude, because of the belief in punishment in the afterlife, was able to state that homosexuals could look forward to eternal punishment in the fires of hell.

It is not surprising to find that New Testament writers were as opposed to homosexuality as writers in the Old Testament, because Christianity developed out of Judaism. The first Christians, including Jesus' disciples and the later followers, such as the apostle Paul, were Jews who brought Jewish beliefs and mindsets into the emerging religion. Jewish scriptures were mined for proof-texts to "prove" that Jesus was the predicted Messiah (cf. Matthew). Jewish food laws and the practice of circumcision were considered by some Christians to be essential to the new faith, while others found these same issues to be peripheral (cf. Galatians).

When Paul and others carried the gospel beyond Palestine to other parts of the Greco-Roman world, they were confronted by sexual mores that they found shocking and in direct violation of the revealed rules found in Jewish scriptures. Certainly among the upper class in Roman and Greek cities (and perhaps also among the poorer people) homosexuality was acceptable.[8] Some Corinthian Christians had been homosexuals but were no longer because of Paul's preaching (1 Cor. 6:11). The implication is clear: to become Christian, homosexuals had to forsake their life-style; Christian faith could "cure" homosexuals.

Homosexuality and the Bible in the Twentieth Century

Attitudes based on biblical teaching continue to affect the lives of homosexuals. Some church groups have refused certain posts within the church structure to homosexuals. A few religious groups, including the Unitarian Universalists and the United Church of Christ, have ordained homosexual pastors (1972). In 1977, the Episcopal church ordained a lesbian. Some groups, such as the American Humanist Association and the American Ethical Union, have no regulations concerning sexual preference for membership or leadership. A number of "gay" groups have been formed within churches. For example, some gay Roman Catholics have grouped together under the title "Dignity"; there is a Jewish gay group called "Achvah"; and there are gay Episcopalian and gay Lutheran groups, and so on. Most are not recognized as "official" in the church or synagogue despite the fact that they advertise their religious affiliations. The metropolitan community churches are composed largely of lesbians, male homosexuals, and those whose sexual interests include both men and women, and the pastors are homosexuals.

Even outside the organized religious community, homosexuals often feel the impact of biblical attitudes. Homosexual teachers and student counselors feel pressured to conceal their sexual preferences and to associate with lovers in secret. Courses in human sexuality and programs in women's studies in colleges and universities have been attacked by members of religious groups in the community for emphasizing the acceptability of male homosexuality and lesbianism.

Few pause to remember that the biblical responses to homosexuality come from Jews and Christians who lived in a small corner of the Mediterranean world two or three thousand years ago. Their beliefs in revealed or inspired revelations of the divine reflect not only their particular sexual biases but the world-view of their time (for example, the three-tiered world of heaven, earth, and hell). Their beliefs were not necessarily those of the wider society of the world, and it is clear from both biblical literature and nonbiblical writings of the same era that there were advanced civilizations (Egyptian, Canaanite, Greek, and Roman) that entertained different attitudes toward homosexuality. The world was then, as it is now, religiously pluralistic. The religious beliefs of one group were authoritative only for that group. Just as in our present pluralistic world, there were varying religious belief-systems and differing attitudes toward homosexuality. Dangerous restrictions of freedoms and rights of minorities occur when the archaic beliefs of one religious group are imposed upon those who hold different interpretations of those beliefs or who may reject them outright. Fortunately, there are within the Western world devout Christians and Jews who place greater emphasis on love and justice and freedom than upon the authority of the handful of biblical passages denegrating homosexuality. Some question the selection of these particular passages from biblical literature by those who conveniently ignore other regulations (such as those pertaining to menstrual uncleanness and divorce). When attempts are made to limit by legislation the ways in which homosexuals can interact in various fields of employment (including public education, recreation, and school counseling), the infringement upon human rights and freedoms begins to reflect totalitarianism.

Comments by the apostle Paul in the Corinthian correspondence suggesting that, when an individual converts to Christianity, sexual preferences become "normal" have helped to shape attitudes toward homosexuality. Homosexual Christians who do not develop heterosexual interests are often made to feel that somehow their beliefs are inadequate and that if only they would "truly accept Christ" they would have the "stigma" removed. There is an implicit denial of the reality that some individuals appear to be born with homosexual tendencies and that there is evidence of some sort of genetic heritage involved. Further, the guilt can spill over to the parents, who ask, "What have I done wrong that my daughter is a lesbian?" or " . . . my son is a homosexual?" Some therapists have attempted to trace sexual preferences back to childhood experiences, to the roles played by parents, and so on, and many suggest that the individual can be changed through faith or therapy and made "normal." The individual is most often ignored and lesbians and male homosexuals are made to feel that they are sinners or "queer."

Homosexuality and Guilt

Few stop to ponder the burden of guilt at not being "normal" that society can place upon the homosexual. The little boy who enjoys arranging the hair on his sister's dolls and who carefully combs and dresses his sister's hair while other boys are out playing ball is called a "sissy." He is made to feel that he is something less than a man and that he is failing to be what he ought to be.

The little girl who loves baseball and who dreams of playing for the Giants or Dodgers when she "grows up" is accepted for a time as a "tomboy" but then discovers that she is growing away from her female playmates. While other girls are content to watch and applaud the boys in their sports, she wants to be involved and to compete. They spend time preparing their bodies and faces for dates; she concentrates on improving her stance at bat. She finds herself more and more isolated and is compelled to seek association with other women who, like her, discover that they are "different." She may be familiar with the term "lesbian" but feels uneasiness in associating it with herself. She may feel she is a failure because she does not measure up to the image of what others believe a woman should be.

Feelings of failure to meet standards accepted as normal, right, and proper by others produce guilt. What can be wrong with a boy who appears to be out of step in developing the accepted male patterns his comrades do. How long is a girl going to be accepted as a tomboy? When does she become a "young lady"?

Among some religious groups there is little tolerance of homosexuals. For example, a young man is a Mormon, has been a missionary for the church, and has received the all-important "patriarchal blessing" in which he is told of a promising future if he continues in the faith. As a "normal" Mormon, he would marry and have a family, but his sexual preference is men. What can he do? He can marry, father several children, and have "affairs" with males on the side and feel dishonest. He can marry, become a parent, and then divorce his wife and feel that he has acted, at least in part, as a "normal" human being. He can fight his feelings and try to make the best of a miserable situation, realizing that as his sexual disinterest in his wife grows stronger—she begins to wonder, "What is wrong with me?"—he has placed a special burden of self-doubt on her.

The same pattern of problems can be found in Roman Catholicism, in Judaism, and in conservative Protestant Christianity. Therapists who work within the settings of their respective denominations are often in a quandary. They can confront the pain experienced by their clients but are in no position to relieve the guilt or provide means for acceptance. The patient is left with a decision: to accept the way of the faith or to go it alone with one's feelings and conscience; there is no way to bring the two together. Those who leave the religion they were raised in may not feel comfortable in a group that does not accept the Bible or church dogma as authoritative and that emphasizes self-fulfillment and personal growth. With all of the pressures that come upon gays from society in general, and sometimes also from the family and church or synagogue, it is not surprising to find a high incidence of suicide among them. The struggle to conform, the feelings of being a failure, of being inadequate, or of being sinful become so burdensome that life does not seem worth continuing.

It was not until December 15, 1973, that the American Psychiatric Association, by formal action, removed homosexuality from its official list of mental disorders. The American Psychological Association took similar action in January 1975. As early as 1953, F. J. Kallman had presented evidence that one factor in the development of homosexual tendencies was genetically determined.[9] The research by Kinsey and his associates found that males who between adolescence and old age had experienced homosexual contacts that culminated in orgasm constituted 37 percent of the male population, and that only 4 percent remained exclusively homosexual throughout their lives.[10] The percentage for females was 13 percent.[11]

It took time for therapists to alter their evaluation of homosexuality, and there are still those who have difficulty in overcoming their personal homophobia when counseling gays or lesbians. Whether the more orthodox religions will be able to give homosexuals full acceptance is yet to be seen. It has been pointed out, for example, that the Mormon church recently accepted blacks into the Levitical priesthood for the first time when a revelation was received in the Upper Room by the church president. Whether a revelation concerning homosexuals will be forthcoming cannot be determined, nor can the future position of the Roman Catholic church. Orthodox Protestant churches and Jewish synagogues are most resistant. The more liberal Protestant churches continue to wrestle with the issue, yielding little by little to acceptance of homosexuals. Meanwhile, the Bible will continue to be used as a religious and social weapon in the attacks on gays and lesbians.

Sodomy

Sodomy, or buggery, refers to anal intercourse. The male inserts his penis into the anus of his partner, who may be either male or female. The insertion of a finger or fingers into the anal passage is a fairly common gesture during lovemaking by lesbians, gays, and heterosexuals. It constitutes a recognition of the anus as an erogenous zone. But this act is not sodomy.

Sodomy is condemned as an unnatural sexual act in the King James translation of the Jewish scriptures. The basic text is Deuteronomy 23:17:

> There shall be no whore [*qedeshah*] of the daughters of Israel nor a sodomite [*qadesh*] of the sons of Israel.

The words *qedeshah* and *qadesh* are derived from a root meaning "to be holy" (*q-d-sh*) and refer to persons engaged in the service of a deity. Modern translations use the more accurate designation of "male cult-prostitute" and "female cult-prostitute." The term *sodomite* does not occur in the Jewish scriptures.

Within the Christian scriptures the term *arsenokoitai* is used to refer to sodomites (1 Cor. 6:9; 1 Tim. 1:10) and means "those who enter the buttocks" and generally is used with reference to a homosexual act. However, as we have noted above, anal intercourse may be performed with a woman as a partner, and is therefore not limited to homosexuals. Homosexuality, like heterosexuality, appreciates the total body of the loved person in lovemaking. What is done, including touching, kissing, fondling, penetration and being penetrated by fingers, tongue, or penis depends upon the tastes, interests, and feeling of comfort of the lovers. To use the term *sodomy* only with reference to homosexuality is to be out of touch with the variety of human sexual activities.

NOTES

1. John Boswell, *Christianity, Social Tolerance, and Homosexuality* (Chicago, 1980); Michael Goodrich, *The Unmentionable Vice: Homosexuality in the Later Medieval Period* (Ross-Erickson, 1979).

2. Leland E. Hinsie and Robert J. Campbell, *Psychiatric Dictionary* (New York, 1960).

3. Don Clark, *Loving Someone Gay* (Millbrae, Calif., 1977), p. 3.

4. R. H. Charles, *The Revelation of St. John* (International Critical Commentary) (New York, 1920), vol. 2, p. 178. In a commentary on Revelation 22:15, where the term *dog* (Greek: *kunes*) is used, Charles notes that "according to the inscription in the temple of Astarte at Larnaka, 'dog' and *qadesh* are linked." In other words, Deuteronomy may be reflecting standard usage.

5. Anthony Phillips, *Deuteronomy* (The Cambridge Bible Commentary on the New English Bible) (Cambridge, 1973), p. 157. Phillips suggests that the term *dog* may not be derogatory, but "indicates . . . a relationship of humble service . . . on behalf of his god."

6. The administrative texts found in the excavation of ancient Ugarit, a Canaanite site, list such sacred persons without indicating functions.

7. In one of the comments about John the Baptist attributed to Jesus, Jesus asks his audience, "What did you go out in the wilderness to see? . . . a man [effeminate man: *malaka*] clothed in soft raiment?" (See also Luke 7:25.) Was John the Baptizer a homosexual?

8. For a discussion of sexual practices and, in particular, homosexuality in the Greco-Roman world, see Otto Kiefer, *Sexual Life in Ancient Rome* (London, 1934); E. Royston Park, *Love in Ancient Rome* (London, 1965), pp. 243 ff.; Hans Licht, *Sexual Life in Ancient Greece* (London, 1932), pp. 411 ff.

9. F. J. Kallmann, *Heredity in Health and Mental Disorder* (New York, 1953).

10. A. C. Kinsey, W. B. Pomeroy, C. E. Martin, *Sexual Behavior in the Human Male* (Philadelphia, 1948).

11. A. C. Kinsey, W. B. Pomeroy, C. E. Martin, *Sexual Behavior in Human Females* (Philadelphia, 1953).

23

Transvestism

A transvestite is one who dresses in the clothing of the opposite sex. Many modern psychologists and psychiatrists view this practice as a sexual deviation; the writer of the book of Deuteronomy labeled it an abomination. The passage is an interesting one:

> A female shall not wear a male's garment, and a male shall not don a female's garment (Deut. 22:5).

The Hebrew word that is translated to "male" here usually designates a warrior or a strong man and the word that is translated to "garment" can be used with reference to a warrior's weapon—his sword, for instance. There were strong taboos in ancient Israel about the association of anything feminine with the warrior. When David's soldier Uriah returned from the battlefield, David hoped that the man would go to his home and have sexual intercourse with his (Uriah's) wife, who was pregnant because of her adulterous affair with David. Uriah was a loyal soldier. He did not go home; he slept in the barracks. To have had intercourse with his wife might have contaminated him or weakened him for battle (2 Sam. 11). So powerful was the taboo against anything sexual being associated with battles or war that even a soldier who had a nocturnal emission was required to leave the encampment for an entire day. He had to perform cleansing rites to remove the pollution associated with the semen (Deut. 23:10). When the Hebrews went to war, they carried with them the sacred ark of Yahweh to signify the presence of their deity in the battle. Because Yahweh was offended by sexual pollution, the nocturnal emission or the presence of one who had engaged in sexual intercourse might cause the withdrawal of divine strength.

It has been suggested that the transvestite prohibition might be directed against participation in customs practiced in the Canaanite religion. In one Canaanite myth, the heroine Paghat donned a warrior's garb to avenge the death of her brother.[1] However, this one reference is not really enough to prove anything about Canaanite religious customs.

In some religions in the ancient Near East and in the Mediterranean world, such as in the cult of Dionysius and in the worship of Astarte, men donned female costumes in the service of the deity, particularly in those instances where, in the mantic frenzy of devotion, the men cut off their genitals as offerings to the goddess.[2] As castrates they wore female clothing.

We cannot know for sure what lay behind the Hebrew law, but the taboo remains as a part of our culture. In the commentary on the Book of Deuteronomy in the Interpreter's Bible, the writers of the homiletic section stated:

> The impersonation of the opposite sex is usually for vulgar and lewd entertainment. In heathenism such exchange of garments was generally for immoral purposes.[3]

Most clergy tend to accept the taboo against transvestites and condemn it as some kind of immoral act or as an unacceptable sexual practice.

Therapists have come to recognize different levels of transvestite behavior or differing patterns in cross-dressing. There are men and women who limit the wearing of the attire of the opposite sex to the privacy of their own homes. Some couples use it as a stimulating deviation in sex behavior and enjoy playing the roles of the opposite sex and even fashion games to go with it. Cross-dressing for these people can be a form of sex play that adds variety to their mutual sexual enjoyment, but their behavior is not public knowledge.

The most apparent examples of cross-dressing can be observed in homosexual gatherings, where "going in drag" is not uncommon. Men who are called "queens" wear female clothing, makeup, and wigs and affect feminine gestures and posture in public places. Some are able to pass as women. Women in male garb are often called "dykes." They can usually be identified as females but act out the accepted male protective role with their women friends.

Some transvestites are stage personalities. Danny Larue (no relative) was a stage attraction in Picadilly, London, for many years, playing to packed houses. Everyone knew he was a man in woman's clothing. He was a professional entertainer. When the comedian Flip Wilson dons women's clothes on the television screen, he does it to provoke laughter.

There are other transvestites who feel more comfortable in the clothing of the opposite sex. The man acts as though he feels that he is a woman with a penis. Some men masturbate when they cross-dress. Some use their cross-dressing experiences as stimulants to heterosexual intercourse. Many are deeply troubled by their behavior and seek counseling. Psychologists use varying kinds of treatment, ranging from mild shock to other forms of aversion therapy, to move the individual away from this behavior. Reasonable success has been reported. None of these individuals want to change their sex. Indeed it has been suggested that the male who cross-dresses feels both an identity with women and a hostility toward them. The female who cross-dresses does not want to become a male but does want to feel more masculine.

There are some psychologists (Jungian) who believe that each of us has within us both a female (anima) and a male (animus) dimension to the personality. Those who cross-dress may be responding to deeply felt needs to respond to the opposite side of their biological self.

Transsexuals

A far more complex dimension of the transvestite issue involves those individuals who feel they are men trapped inside of women's bodies or women in men's bodies. They seek transsexual operations to enable them to feel that they are what they were meant to be.

The problem of gender identity begins at a very young age and may be manifested first in something as simple as the desire of a two-year-old to dress up in the clothing of the opposite sex, perhaps only to play "Daddy" or "Mommy." Some have argued that the gender-identity problem may be genetically determined or represent some pattern of fetal growth or some chromosome variation. Others suggest that a number of factors, particularly early infant and childhood experiences, are determinants.[4]

No matter what the causes of problems of gender identification may be, some individuals have operations to change their genital structure. Males are treated with hormones to increase breast size and with electrolysis to remove facial hair, and they have their penis and testicles removed and a vagina constructed by a plastic surgeon, who thrusts the penis sheath into the body cavity. The results are often startling and these men-become-women are accepted as women. They date, they marry, they have sexual intercourse with men and sometimes are able to achieve orgasm. The change of a woman into a man is more complex. Breasts are removed by mastectomy, the uterus and inner female organs are taken out by a panhysterectomy. Male characteristics, including facial hair, are encouraged with testosterone. So far, it has not been possible for plastic surgeons to provide a functioning penis and testes. A penis is formed from body skin and flesh, usually taken from the abdomen. A penis implant provides enough rigidity for intercourse. Orgasmic response depends entirely upon what the surgeon does to the clitoris, which can be repositioned to enable the person to experience a sexual climax. There is, of course, no ejaculation.

It should not be assumed that anatomical changes are made casually. Before accepting a patient for such an operation, the plastic surgeon requires the person to submit to a battery of psychological tests and interviews to determine the depth of the feeling of being a person of a different sex in the wrong body. Post-surgical counseling is also important because the adjustment period can be harrowing. The greater the acceptance of the "new" person by friends and family, the greater the ease in moving into the new role.

Sometimes there is a need to prove or demonstrate or reenforce the feelings of a new sexual identity. Some transsexuals become prostitutes for short periods of time. Sometimes prostitution becomes a means of economic survival during the transition period, while the acquisition of a new identity with new personal documents and credentials is under way. Most would prefer to prove sexual identity by marriage. The physical changes are usually so complete and so well done that the person has no difficulty in passing as a naturally born member of the sex chosen. Exact figures of the number of successful transsexual operations are hard to estimate, but such procedures are more numerous than most imagine and have been estimated in the thousands.

The responses to transsexuals by religious groups varies. Orthodox Christians and Jews condemn sex changes. If biblical proof-texts are needed, the Deuteronomic ruling is cited and reinforced by arguments to the effect that humans should not play God by changing their natural state into something that is unnatural. The liberal groups that do not use the Bible as a guide for ethics and morals suggest that what appears to be right for specific individuals and what seems to enhance their lives or free them for greater creative enjoyment should be accepted—after all, they are not harming anyone.

NOTES

1. Theodor H. Gaster, *Thespis, Ritual, Myth and Drama in the Ancient Near East* (New York, 1950, 1961), p. 373.

2. Cf. Theodor H. Gaster, *Myth, Legend and Custom in the Old Testament.* (New York, 1969, 1975), vol. 1, pp. 316 ff.

3. Henry H. Shires and Pierson Parker, "The Book of Deuteronomy: Exposition," *The Interpreter's Bible* (New York, Nashville, 1953), vol. 2, pp. 464 f.

4. For a clear discussion, see Robert J. Stoller, "Gender Identity," in Benjamin J. Sadock, Harold I. Kaplan, and Alfred M. Freedman, eds., *The Sexual Experience* (Baltimore, 1976), pp. 182–196. For a transsexual's personal story that parallels much of what Stoller reports, see Canary Conn, *Canary: The Story of a Transsexual* (Los Angeles, 1974).

24

Masturbation

Attitudes toward masturbation have varied from culture to culture. In the ancient Near East, differing attitudes seem to have prevailed. For example, in certain Egyptian creation myths the god created by means of masturbation. The Shabaka stone, which is now in the British museum, tells of the sun-god Atum, whose cult center was at On (Heliopolis), who brought everything into being "through his semen and his fingers." The late-fourth-century B.C.E. Bremner-Rhinds Papyrus (also in the British Museum) records statements attributed to the sun-god Ra-Atum: "I was the one who with my fist stimulated desire; I masturbated with my hand and I spat it [the semen] from my mouth . . ." and the expectorated semen was the stuff of creation.

What was acceptable for the gods may not have been acceptable for humans. There can be little doubt that, in the miming or reenacting of the myths, what the gods did in the beginning, the priests did in ritual. That is, within the cultus, the act of masturbation, the taking of the semen into the mouth, and the spitting forth of the semen would be done by the priests. But temple precincts are sacred territory and what was done in ritual might not be done outside of it. The famous negative confession in the Egyptian Book of the Dead provides the dead pharaoh with the words he must speak in the hall of judgment to be able to pass on to eternal bliss. He is to state: "I have not masturbated in the temples of my city god." Whether the pharaoh masturbated in the creation rituals in the temple precincts of the supreme god Atum, we cannot know. Nor do we know if the pharaoh masturbated when he was not in the temple precincts of the city god. So far as we can tell there was no prohibition against masturbation per se by the general populace.

Nor is there any clear-cut evidence relating to attitudes toward masturbation in Mesopotamian cultures. Other sexual practices are mentioned, so that one can assume that masturbation was also practiced and that there was no specific prohibition.

There is no legislation pertaining to masturbation in the Bible. One possible reference is in the story of Onan (Gen. 38), but Onan's "sin" has been interpreted both as masturbation and as coitus interruptus (withdrawal before ejaculation). The story is actually a bit of Hebrew folklore related to the ancient custom of levirate or brother-in-law marriage. When a married man died without offspring, it was the duty of the next-of-kin to have sexual intercourse with the dead man's wife to provide a son to carry on the dead man's name. At this time, immortality appears to have been thought of as continuation of the name of the deceased male in the offspring who would preserve the family line. Legal details are spelled out in Deuteronomy 25:5ff. The story of Ruth is also related to this custom. (See "The Levirate," Chapter 3.)

In the Genesis story, Er, the son of Judah, married Tamar, but before she could become pregnant Er offended Yahweh and the deity killed him. It was now up to Onan to fulfill the levirate requirements. But, whenever he went into his brother's wife, Onan, knowing that the seed (child) would not be reckoned as his, ejaculated on the ground ("destroyed his semen on the ground"), thereby depriving his brother of offspring. This was offensive to the deity, so Yahweh killed him too. The story goes on to tell how Tamar tricked her father-in-law into having intercourse with her to provide offspring for Judah's dead son Er.

We are not told exactly what Onan did. Was it coitus interruptus or masturbation? Many commentators suggest that it was the former, but there has been a long-standing belief among Jews and Christians that Onan masturbated. In either case, the act was offensive to the deity, and what the god rejects his followers, in particular the clergy, must oppose. It is not surprising that English-language dictionaries explain the term *onanism* as either masturbation or coitus interruptus. The modern Hebrew term for "masturbation" is *onanuth*, the verb "to masturbate" is *ma'aseh onan* and a masturbator is an *onan*.

There is perhaps one other Bible reference to masturbation. In the collection of sayings attributed to Jesus in the Gospel of Matthew (the so-called Sermon on the Mount) one group of sayings has to do with sexual impurity. Adultery and lustful thoughts are condemned. Then Jesus added: "And if your right hand causes you to sin, cut it off and throw it away! It is better to lose one of your members than your whole body should be cast into Gehenna" (Matt. 5:30). The passage follows a saying that, if the eye offends with lustful glances, it should be removed; but there is no way that the hand can be linked to the sayings that preceded it, unless Jesus is referring to the Jewish taboo against masturbation. If so, then here, as in other requirements, he goes beyond Jewish law in his overdramatic call for amputation.

Modern religious taboos against masturbation seem to be a strange mixture of religious belief and folklore. The religious dimensions appear in the arguments that sex is somehow "sacred," that sexual relations are primarily, if not solely, for procreation and that masturbation is a wasting of "seed" that was designed for procreation, thereby thwarting the divine purpose. Moreover, self-stimulation, self-enjoyment in the act of masturbation, is selfish and an act of self-love as well as a misuse of the body. Indeed, there was a time within Roman Catholicism when masturbation was labeled "self-abuse," and little boys entering the confessional were expected to inform the listening priest "how many times" they had performed this act, so that the penance would fit the sin.

Where did the synagogue and the church find the biblical basis for the condemnation of masturbation as a sin? From the story of Onan, and because Onan's sin represented unacceptable sexual behavior to Jews and Christians, children in Western cultures have been raised to believe that masturbation is not only a sin against God but is somehow unclean. One young man recalled that, when he was six years old, his mother told him always to pull back the foreskin (he was uncircumcised) and wash behind the glans as part of his bathing. The boy discovered that the sensation was pleasant and began to masturbate. Only when he was older did he realize that this was what was called "masturbation," which was forbidden by the Mormon church, to which he belonged. The rules of the church had come into conflict with the impulses of the body and began a conflict of emotions that occurred every time he yielded to his bodily feelings.

Little children, who explore their bodies as naturally as they investigate everything else in their environment in their quest to understand their world, have their attention directed away from their genitals. They are told they "must not touch" or that it is "not nice" or perhaps "dirty" to fondle themselves. Folkloric interpretations are added, and for generations boys (and sometimes girls) were told that if they masturbated they would get warts or grow hair on the palms of their hands. One young man recalled: "When I was twelve, I got warts all over my hands. The Methodist minister told my friends not to play with me because I was a sinner."

The religious prohibition was supported by "scientific" observations.[1] In 1774, S. A. D. Tissot wrote a book in French that was translated into English and published in 1832 under the title *Onana: Treatise on the Diseases Produced by Onanism*. It became a basic text for subsequent writings on the subject of masturbation. Tissot equated the loss of a single ounce of seminal fluid with the loss of more than forty ounces of blood, and related gonorrhea, dropsy, and consumption to masturbation. In 1838, Dr. M. S. Gove published a volume called *Solitary Vice*, which persuaded some physicians that masturbation could lead to insanity.

Others added to the list of disorders supposedly stemming from masturbation. For females, there were displacement of the uterus, various menstrual difficulties, hysteria, catalepsy, mental disorders, and so on. For both sexes there were warnings that masturbation could produce dementia, imbecility, and other mental imbalances. Masturbation was said to affect memory, to affect the power of association, and to produce laziness. Masturbators would become gloomy, sullen, irritable, morose and taciturn, embarrassed and awkward, avoiding eye contact and without any energy for the usual pleasures of life. The genitals were said to be affected with abnormal growth and appearance. Essays were written on the causes of masturbation, which included everything from climate, social habits (dancing and riding), economic factors (rich people were idle), intellectual and moral causes (too much study of the fine arts and their lascivious pictures), religious causes (too great a curiosity by the confessor in the confessional) plus a number of general causes, such as impotence in a spouse, and so on.

Some managed to outgrow the folkloric and pseudoscientific warnings; others, particularly those whose belief-systems still emphasized the "evils" of masturbation, continued to experience feelings of guilt, shame, and sinfulness.

On a religious call-in talk-show, a male caller asked the priest on the panel for guidance. He was a Catholic. To date he and his wife had been unable to produce a child. His doctor had suggested a sperm count and asked for a sample of his semen, which would require a masturbatory act. The priest, more liberal than some, suggested he go along with his doctor. "But," the man replied, "my parish priest tells me the opposite and says that even masturbating for a sperm count is a sin. What do I do?" The priest explained that the problem was "pleasure" and that masturbation as "total self-pleasure" was wrong because it was "selfish." The man had already resolved his dilemma. He had decided to "go with the doctor" and, having found that masturbation was a pleasant experience, decided also to go with his feelings! When the show was off the air, the priest commented: "What guilt we produce in people."

Feelings of disgust, generated by being taught that the vagina is not a clean organ, have resulted in some women's inability to experience orgasm,[2] and have educated some women to approach sex with feelings of uncertainty and with a sense of being somehow tainted. Men, too, educated in religious traditions that taught that masturbation was sinful and injurious to health, wrestled with the dilemma of feelings of guilt and fear of offending the deity in conflict with their natural sexual impulses.

Present-day sex studies have demonstrated that masturbation is normal—and harmless. Most liberal clergy have accepted these findings, but some, steeped in the traditions of the past and fearful of sex education, reject the modern findings and cling to old concepts, continuing to generate guilt and the sense of being unworthy in the eyes of the deity in those who respond to normal, natural body feelings.

NOTES

1. Eduard Lea, "The 'Monster Hideous in Mien,' " in *Sexual Self-Stimulation*, ed. by R. E. L. Masters (Los Angeles, 1967), pp. 22–31; Jacobus Sutor, "Onanism in Women," ibid., pp. 52–68; Lester W. Dearborn, "Masturbation" in *Human Autoerotic Practices*, ed. by Manfred F. DeMartino (New York, 1979), pp. 36–53.

2. See Lonnie Garfield Barbach, *For Yourself* (New York, 1975), pp. 10, 20 ff.

25

Fantasy

One of the "evils" often associated with masturbation is the indulgence in lustful imagery. What do masturbators think about while they are caressing themselves? What do they fantasize? Do they personalize their self-stimulation by imagining they are engaging in coitus with another person? Or do they simply focus on the enjoyment of body sensations without introducing some imaginary event or person? If they do fantasize, is the fantasizing dangerous or evil?

Studies have shown that for some persons masturbation is enjoyed for the physical experience alone. For example, very young children who have no information about sexual relations with another person enjoy the feelings produced by self-caressing. They caress themselves because it feels pleasant, and sometimes they do it almost absent-mindedly while looking at a picture book. Some children learn at an early age to play with another child's genitals.[1] Their mental imaging at this stage may be related to a partial distortion of what birth and reproduction are all about, or it may be a mental expression, with physical accompaniments, of the need for tender parenting.[2]

In adolescence, fantasizing during masturbation becomes almost commonplace. It has been reported that "only 11 percent of the boys and 7 percent of the girls who are currently masturbating say they never daydream or fantasize during masturbation."[3] Boys appear to daydream more often than girls. Images produced by boys include sex with someone forced to submit, sex with more than one female, group sex, sex when he himself is forced to submit, sex with varying degrees of violence toward the other person, and oral and anal sex. Girls' fantasies are often about sex with a much admired male, sex with more than one male when the girl is forced to submit, sex with mild violence inflicted on the other person, and passive oral sex.[4] For some adolescents, masturbation and masturbatory imagery can become a source of internal conflict due to guilt. Adolescents may wonder if they are developing normally or whether such imaging is abnormal. They may feel that they are coming under the control of urges and drives from which there is no escape.[5]

In Hebrew thinking, as in the thinking of others in the ancient world, the heart was believed to be the center of the intellect. A worshiper could ask the deity to "incline my heart to thy testimonies" (Ps. 119:36), meaning turn my thoughts or my mind toward your teachings. In the King James version of the Bible, Proverbs 23:7 was translated "For as he thinketh in his heart so is he," a translation that is no longer accepted as accurate. Nevertheless the idea has not lost its potency because of new translations. For many, the inward thought is betrayal of true intent, true desire, and indeed may be the beginning of some act. Thus, for some, what one fantasizes reveals what the person is in reality.

Some fantasizing takes place during sexual intercourse. The person may imagine they are making love to someone other than their partner—a screen star or some other person of the same or opposite sex, or even with an animal. Some feel that the fantasizing is important in reaching climax, some believe it adds an element of excitement and variation to coitus.

Some partners are able to share their fantasies, others are not. Some find it very threatening to discover that their partner is not thinking about what is being shared but is actually embracing another person. Questions come to mind: "What is the matter with me that she [or he] finds it necessary to imagine that I am someone else?" "Am I an inadequate or unsatisfactory sexual partner?" "What has she [or he] got that I haven't got?" The result can be a negative self-examination that can seriously affect the nourishing aspects of lovemaking.

Some people become very angry. "How dare he use me to fulfill his desire to be with so-and-so?" "I feel really put down and used as a sexual object!" "This dirty so-and-so is not interested in me as a person or a lover, but is just relieving sexual tension while mooning over someone else!"

Some feel betrayed. "I thought we had a special bond between us, but now it is as though he were sleeping with someone else." "I thought she was in love with me, but obviously this is not so. She is really attracted to another." "Clearly this marks the end of our relationship. If I am not good enough for him then let him go and be with the person he desires."

Many therapists point out that fantasizing during masturbation or coitus is not abnormal. Sharing the fantasy with one's lover is acceptable only if it is not threatening to the relationship. They do not condemn what they accept as a rather common happening, but they are sensitive to the ways in which acknowledging the fantasy can threaten a relationship. They draw sharp distinctions between what is imagined and what is actualized and point to the gulf between the thought and the deed. In private sessions with an individual, they probe the basis for the fantasy and its meaning for the individual's personal health and development. In family sessions, they may consider it wise not to open the subject for discussion.

Not all therapists agree that fantasizing during the sexual act is normal or acceptable. Freud provided a basis for their objections when he stated that "happy people never make fantasies, only unsatisfied ones."[6] Some of Freud's followers believe that fantasies engaged in during intercourse are diversionary tactics to avoid full orgasmic surrender. Women patients more often than men appear to be the target for such a judgment. Barbara Hariton suggested that perhaps this is because "Psychology is dominated by males who find it impossible that normal women might have fantasies during intercourse" and thus sexual fantasies can be described as "tortuous efforts to satisfy other needs through sex, as expressions of penis fear, as devices employed by some women to put psychological distance between themselves and their partners, and as mechanisms to deny responsibility for performing sex acts that would lead to intolerable guilt.'"[7] It is not surprising that "several therapists note that women are reluctant to discuss their sexual fantasies, that they seem to fear disapproval." Theodore Reich stated that fantasies during intercourse occur more often among women than men, basing his claim on "what psychoanalysts know from their psychiatric practice.'"[8] Women who have been victims of incest during childhood report that, because of the trauma of the incest experience, as adults they tend to block all imaging, including fantasizing about their partner during intercourse.

Imaging, the ability or desire to fantasize, varies from person to person and is affected in large measure by past experiences and by the mood or the needs of the moment. To label it "good" or "bad" or "abnormal" is to place moral and psychological judgment on the act and suggest that there is some sort of behavioral aberration in the thought process. It is important to acknowledge that fantasizing during the sexual act is a human reality, that it may or may not signify dissatisfaction with the present partner, that it may or may not be used to enhance a sexual setting, that it may or may not become obsessive or toxic, and that it may or may not be wise to share the fantasy with one's sex partner.

Some couples act out sexual fantasies. They dress in clothing that dramatizes the roles they are playing. They act the way they imagine the screen star or hero-figure might act in the setting. They may pretend that they have just met and this is their first time for intercourse. They may pretend to be male or female prostitutes and rent a hotel room and play out the fantasy to the full. Some declare that sexual intercourse is heightened by the fantasy games; others say that they indulge in them for fun, just as they participate in other activities together for fun. It is really not surprising to find that couples who give the public appearance of being rather staid, proper, and conservative people in their community associations, do, on occasion, escape into the world of sexual fantasy. They rent a room in one of the motels set up for this kind of experience. Walls and ceilings are mirrored. The lighting, controlled by a rheostat, is either soft or bright, depending on their wishes. The room is equipped with a refrigerator and a small stove, so they can warm their food and cool their drinks—or they can have meals delivered to the door and never have to leave their fantasy world. There is soft music or, if they like, a television screen that will bring erotic or pornographic movies into their environment. These outings are kept secret from all but the most understanding friends. They have found a setting that provides them with the maximum opportunity for fantasizing and living out their fantasies.

There are many members of conservative religious groups who find this sort of behavior depraved and obnoxious. They refer to the attitudes toward lust found in the Bible and put this sort of behavior into the category of "perverted" or "animal-like." Some would seek to close down the motels that cater to such outrageous sexual goings-on, despite the fact that many of those who rent the rooms are married couples with families who are seeking an opportunity for privacy, fun, and sexual experimentation with one another. There is a hard line of thinking among some of these ultraconservatives that sex is for procreation, that it should be quiet and discreet, and that probably it should be performed only in the darkness of the night and in "the missionary position." One need only visit Pompeii and the Naples museum to discover that sexual fantasy has been part of the human enjoyment of sex for millennia. One can only ask, "How can what a couple do in the privacy of their own motel room, no matter how lavishly or outrageously that room may be decorated, do any harm to anyone but themselves? And, if they are enjoying themselves, where is the evil?"

NOTES

1. William V. Silverberg, *Childhood Experience and Personal Destiny* (New York, 1952), pp. 162 f.

2. Rose Edgecumbe and Marion Burgner, "The Phallic-Narcissistic Phase," in *The Psychoanalytic Study of the Child* (New Haven, 1975), vol. 30, pp. 166 ff.

3. Robert C. Sorenson, "Various Aspects of Masturbation by Teenage Boys and Girls," in *Human Autoerotic Practices*, ed. by Manfred F. DeMartino (New York, 1979), p. 98.

4. Ibid., p. 99.

5. Stanley H. Shapiro, "Vicissitudes of Adolescence," in *Behavior Pathology of Childhood and Adolescence*, ed. by Sidney L. Copel (New York, 1973), pp. 96 ff.

6. Sigmund Freud, *Delusions and Dreams* (Boston, 1956), p. 126.

7. E. Barbara Hariton, "The Sexual Fantasies of Women," in *Readings in Human Sexuality: Contemporary Perspectives*, ed. by Chad Gordon and Gayle Johnson (New York, 1976), p. 280.

8. Theodore Reich, "The Emotional Differences of the Sexes," in *Of Love and Lust* (New York, 1949), p. 430.

26

Lust

Lust has come to mean sensuous sexual appetite or desire, or to use psychological terminology, "libidinous desire." It is often associated with the idea of "animal passions," which suggests that sexual eagerness is somehow subhuman. Lust in its sexual connotation is considered to be a sin, or a contributing factor to sin, by many religious groups. Lust or desire for something approved of by the religious group, such as lusting after the kingdom of God, is not condemned.

The tenth commandment of the Decalogue forbids coveting the wife of one's neighbor (Exod. 20:17; Deut. 5:21). The woman is listed with other chattels, including the house, the servants, and the livestock. Coveting in this instance does not mean sexual desire, but rather is related to desire for the acquisition of valuable property belonging to another male. It could be translated "You shall not be greedy for . . ." Covetousness has to do with desire for material possessions, which can be the fantasy of a lazy man who sits back and feeds his hunger for things in daydreams but fails to perform the labor necessary to acquire them (Prov. 21:25).

In the Jewish scriptures, lust is most often applied to the nation Israel in prophetic condemnations that accuse the people of abandoning their god Yahweh in their lusting after what other nations and other gods can offer. The prophet Ezekiel, an exile in Babylon during the sixth century B.C.E., used allegory to depict the relationships of the divided kingdoms of Judah and Israel to their god Yahweh (Ezek. 23). Yahweh (he wrote) married two whores, Olaha (Israel) and Oholibah (Judah). These were women who had been used by the Egyptians, whose breasts had been fondled until their nipples were bruised—not very savory characters! After their marriage to Yahweh (a symbol of becoming Yahweh worshipers), they were not satisfied. Israel lusted after the Assyrians and prostituted herself to them—"in her youth they laid [fornicated] with her, bruisedly handled her virgin breasts and poured their ejaculations upon her" (Ezek. 23:8). The historical fact is that Assyria had conquered Israel in the eighth century and had absorbed the people into the Assyrian empire. Ezekiel claimed that the conquest came because Yahweh was angry at the infidelity of the nation and delivered the people into the hands of the enemy. In other words, the fall of Israel was the will of Yahweh.

Judah, in Ezekiel's mind, was even worse than Israel. Judah had not only become a whore for the Assyrians, but also for the Babylonians. She lusted after and invited "to her bed of love [lust]" her paramours, "whose penises are like the penises of asses" and "whose ejaculations are like the ejaculations of horses" (Ezek. 23:20).

The prophet uses the unfaithful-wife image in describing the divine-human relationships between Yahweh and the City of Jerusalem (Ezek. 16). He describes the origin of the city: It came into being in the land of Canaan as the offspring of an Amorite father and a Hittite mother. The child (city), a female, was unwanted and was exposed to die until it was rescued by Yahweh.[1]

The child grew to young maidenhood. She became tall and fully ripe—"your breasts were firm and your [pubic] hair luxuriant." But she was still nude (16:7). Yahweh knew she had arrived at the time "for love [lust]" and cast his cloak over her—a symbol of protection and sexual possession. Yahweh clothed and beautified Jerusalem, but the city began to solicit the favors of each passer-by like a common whore. The prophetic imagery continues. Jerusalem took the silver and gold lavished on her by Yahweh and converted it into "male images," which may refer to phalli or dildoes used in the fertility cult. Shrines for the fertility religions were erected at the head of every street, and there on couches set before the sacred altars, patrons could engage in intercourse with the cult prostitutes in the name of one divinity or another.

Jerusalem also fornicated with Egypt, the prophet wrote, that neighbor "great of flesh"—a reference to the size of Egyptian penises. So lustful was the city that it engaged in fornication with Assyria and Babylon, while at the same time increasing its sexual intercourse with Canaan. This lustful behavior spelled the doom of Jerusalem. "Because your menstrual discharge was poured out and your vulva was displayed through your whoring with your lovers and with all the idols of your [ritual] abominations" the adulterous city would be destroyed. The punishment came not only because Jerusalem worked as a whore without payment but because it yielded sexually to aliens rather than remaining faithful to Yahweh, the husband.

The allegory of the sacred marriage between the nation of the city of Jerusalem and Yahweh seems to have originated in the eighth century with the prophet Hosea. Hosea's wife, Gomer, became a follower of the Canaanite fertility god Ba'al. As far as Hosea was concerned, Gomer was a symbol of the nation, and the anger and anguish he felt at her betrayal of the marriage bond was what the prophet believed the deity must also be experiencing. He wrote that he married Gomer because Yahweh commanded him, "Go, take for yourself a whorish wife" (Hos. 1:2). Hosea's experience with his whoring wife was a metaphor for Yahweh's experience with the whoring nation.

The sacred marriage motif appears also in Jeremiah (2:1–3; 3:1–5) and in the post-exilic portion of the Book of Isaiah (50:1). The father-son metaphor was also used (cf. Exod. 4:22; Hos. 11:1; Jer. 31:9, 20), but most often the relationship between the god and his people was depicted in ruler-servant terms (Jer. 30:10; Ezek. 28:25; Isa. 41:8–9; 42:1; 43:10, etc.). It is in Ezekiel that the imagery of the unfaithful wife reaches its fullest development.

Ezekiel portrays the foreign lovers as having huge penises and forceful ejaculations. Few scholars care to dwell on this material, and the homiletic material finds the whole scene unappetizing and unfit for public reading. One cannot but wonder what lies behind the descriptions.

Freud described penis-envy as a characteristic of women. "They feel seriously wronged, often declare that they want to 'have something like it too' and fall victim to 'envy for the penis.' "[2] Present-day sex therapists have made other contributions to the concept. Although there may be some fundamental truth in Freud's analysis (and it has been challenged),[3] it has been found that male sexual performance can, at times, be affected by what has been called the "phallic fallacy" or the "penile fallacy," but which is often known in popular jargon as "male penis envy." The problem arises when males become aware of the differences in size between their own and other penises. This awareness, accompanied by folkloric beliefs that the bigger the penis, the more effective the sexual encounter or the better the lover, can produce feelings of inadequacy in some males. Feelings of inadequacy can, in turn, affect the male's ability to achieve or maintain an erection. Indeed, any reference to inferior penis-size by a sex partner may induce temporary impotency. The fallacy lies in the belief that size is a significant factor in satisfactory lovemaking and in the belief that there is a significant difference in the length and circumference of erect penises, which may be distinctly different in size while flaccid. Both fallacies have been put to rest over and over again by sex researchers but continue to circulate nevertheless.[4]

Exactly what Ezekiel was hoping to imply by the references to the size of the non-Hebrew penises is not clear. There can be little question that the fertility cults with their ritual prostitution had an impact on the religion of Yahweh, and the worship of gods and goddesses whose rites included copulation was widespread. All of this is clear from the protests of the prophets, including Hosea, Amos, Jeremiah, and Ezekiel. It is generally assumed that the references to the size of the penis and the force of the ejaculation of foreigners are denigrations, reflecting disgust for those who copulate with the lustful passion of animals in heat (Jer. 2:23–24).

On the other hand, it is possible that phallic imagery was as common in Palestine as it was in Egypt. On the walls of temples and in drawings on papyri and in tomb paintings, the Egyptians portrayed the god Min with his penis hard and erect. The copulation scenes from the Osirian cult dramatize liturgical enactments of mythological accounts in formal temple rituals. Sometimes the male genitals are exaggerated to immense proportions. It is not impossible that some of this imagery was present in the street shrines condemned by Ezekiel. Among cultic objects found in excavations in Palestine, in addition to plaques depicting the nude fertility goddess and female figurines with the large breasts of the *dea nutrix* (nursing mother) type, clay phalli have been found. Further excavation may add more information.

Perhaps Ezekiel is reporting a physical reality that he has somehow been made aware of. Perhaps the foreigners did have larger penises after which the women of Jerusalem lusted, thus giving the metaphor of the nation lusting after foreign gods some basis in fact. Perhaps, too, the prophet was declaring that sex with the foreigners—Egyptians, Assyrians, and Babylonians—was the equivalent of having intercourse with animals, an act of bestiality that was condemned in Jewish law.

Lust in Christian Scriptures

In Christian scriptures lust refers to sexual passions, erotic desires, and also the hunger for the pleasures of the world. Jesus is reported to have said that "whoever looks at a woman lustfully has already committed adultery with her" (Matt. 5:28)—a comment that parallels a saying found in the *Discourses* of Epictetus, who also lived in the first century C.E. Epictetus wrote, "Everyone who looks at a women [lustfully] is as though he had lain with her" (II.18.15).[5] The idea that the thought is the equivalent of the deed and that lust equals fornication is not uniquely Christian. But Epictetus does not affect our world, the Christian teaching does.

The idea is extreme, as many of Jesus' sayings were. Milo Connick has commented:

> What is the lustful look? It is persistent purposing. It is not the consummation (adultery) or the consideration (glance, thought, desire) but the commitment (conscious choice, will). According to Moses, a man alone on an island could not commit adultery. Jesus said he could, if his persistent purpose was to treat a woman as a passing pleasure rather than a person. No woman need be present for a man to commit adultery with her in his heart.[6]

For many the whole idea is unreasonable. To think is not to perform; to dream is not to fulfill; to want or desire is not to acquire. If it were otherwise, then every daydream of robbing a bank and getting away with it, or taking another's Maseratti without paying for it, and every wish in anger for the power to knock someone down and pound one's own wisdom into him would be grounds for criminal action. Adultery is an act, not a fantasy. Unlike Professor Connick, many Christians do not distinguish between his neat categories of "glance, thought, desire" and "conscious choice, will." Nor does the New Testament make these distinctions. For many, perhaps for most believers, the passage means exactly what it says: to look at a woman lustfully is, in the eyes of Jesus and presumably of God, the equivalent of committing adultery with her. It was this interpretation that seems to have been in the mind of President Jimmy Carter when he admitted that he had been guilty of lustful thoughts.

For the believer, the result of accepting this teaching as a divinely revealed regulation is guilt. Not everyone is able to sublimate thinking to the extent that lustful thoughts never become part of the thought process. Even the monastics who renounced the world and its evils continued to struggle with sexual fantasies. The Roman Catholic church provides the confessional to relieve the feelings of guilt in a believer who violates Jesus' teaching. The priest assigns an appropriate act of penance to expiate the sin and the believer promises to try not to commit the sin again. Within some evangelical Protestant communities, public profession of sin is practiced and individuals state their transgressions before the congregation. Most Protestant churches have no means of alleviating the guilt feelings in those who commit inner and secret violations of this lust ruling. The most guilt-filled appear to be adolescents who are coming into sexual maturation. They ask, "Does it count if you find yourself becoming sexually aroused when you are on the beach where there is a girl wearing a string bikini and almost everything she has is hanging out?" "Does it count if you find yourself watching a girl walking down the street and are fascinated by the movement of her hips and think: Wow, I would really like to get into that! Does it count?" And what of the girl who stares at the interesting bulge on the front of the young man's swimming trunks and wonders how it would feel to make out with him? Does it count? In the light of the Christian scriptures, the answer has to be: It does count. And perhaps the "sin" can be broadened to include the glances, whistles, and catcalls that men, young and old, give a shapely woman.

How do those who accept the Christian scriptures as divine revelation and precepts for guidance in life deal with their guilt feelings? Some turn to prayer. "Dear Abby" published a letter from a teen-aged girl who signed it "Walking with God in Bay, Ark." The girl wrote of her fiancé's "test of manhood." "When he is tempted to go beyond a kiss, he has me place my hand beside his on his Bible, and he asks God to give him strength to be the man he needs to be."[7] In other words, this couple finds strength to resist what they must believe are lascivious thoughts and desires that could lead to sexual intercourse by employing prayer and by using the Bible as a talisman. In the words of another couple who also use prayer, they "rise above" lustful thoughts. They set aside their thinking about sex and focus on "spiritual things." They sublimate desire. Others report that they confess their sins to God in private prayer and believe that, having confessed and expressed regret over their sin, they are forgiven. Some carry guilt and are miserable, while still others find a therapist with whom they can share their feelings.

The apostle Paul and other Christian writers in the New Testament emphasize the difference between flesh and spirit, between "things of this world" and those that belong to the world of faith. The use of the terms *flesh* and *fleshy* (*sarx, sarxikos*), while at times appearing to signify sexual desires, often mean "worldly desires.'' Believers are expected to rise above worldly lusts that burden the non-Christians and to focus on the eternal truths of the faith, looking beyond the transient pleasures of the world. Christians are called upon to abandon sexual impulses and desires and to be caught up in the spiritual world of the redeemed. The nature of these desires of the flesh include ''adultery, prostitution, impurity, lewdness, idolatry, sorcery, enmity,'' and so on (Gal. 5:19 f.). The fruits of the spirit are qualities of ''love, joy, peace, patience'' and so on (Gal. 5:22 f.). The sexual aspects of the ways of the world are contrasted to the ways of the faith.

Paul urged members of the Christian group in Thessalonica each to ''achieve mastery over [protect] his member [vessel = genitals], to hallow it and honor it, not in lustful desire like the Gentiles who do not know God'' (1 Thess. 4:4). When he wrote to Christians in Rome, he condemned those who yielded to lustful impulses and who, burning with sexual passion, engaged in homosexual acts (Rom. 1:24–27). He urged Roman Christians, as he did the Thessalonians, ''not to yield to physical desires'' (Rom. 6:12 f.). The same theme appears in Colossians, where the Christians are told to ''kill the earthy impulses [the members which are of the earth] fornication, impurity, lust, evil sexual desire and that avarice which is idolatry'' (Col. 3:5). Beyond the Pauline corpus, 1 Peter 2:11 warns believers against indulging in ''carnal lusts,'' and the admonition is expanded in 2 Peter 2:10–22, where the writer mentions those who ''continually lust after a woman.''

The condemnation of lust in the Christian writings not only produces a sense of guilt in those who experience sexual desire, but also feelings of imperfection in their Christian belief. The results can be traumatic. On the other hand, Christianity assures its followers that such feelings can be overcome and diverted into acceptable and creative channels.

NOTES

1. Exposure of female infants was customary among Arabs until the time of Muhammad, who forbade the practice.

2. Sigmund Freud, *New Introductory Lectures on Psychoanalysis* (New York, 1964), p. 125.

3. Kate Millett, *Sexual Politics* (New York, 1970), pp. 176 ff.

4. Cf. William H. Masters and Virginia E. Johnson, *Human Sexual Response* (Boston, 1966), pp. 191 ff.

5. Quoted by Sherman E. Johnson, ''Matthew: Exegesis,'' *The Interpreter's Bible* (Nashville–New York, 1951), vol. 7, p. 297.

6. Milo Connick, *Jesus: The Man, the Mission and the Message* (New Jersey, 1963), p. 243.

7. The *Los Angeles Times*, June 10, 1982.

27

Dreams

Closely allied with the fantasies that an individual may produce during waking hours are those dreams that come unbidden during sleep. A woman's sexual dreams may cause her vagina to lubricate and can result in an orgasm. There is no physical evidence by which an outsider can know what she has dreamed or experienced in the dream unless she discloses it. But for a man it is quite different. Almost every adolescent boy (and many older men, too) has awakened with an erection. The body is relaxed and the penis responds to whatever the mind generates, or perhaps the mind responds with an image appropriate to the physical impulse. Quite often the erect penis is associated with a full bladder's producing what some have called a ''piss-hard,'' but studies have shown there is no relation between the bladder and the erection.

Sometimes the man awakens to discover that he had ejaculated during sleep. For the youth living at home, there is often some embarrassment associated with the experience. He rises and gets a damp cloth and wipes up the seminal fluid, or he removes his soiled pajamas, folds the sheets over the wet spot and goes back to sleep, or he waits until morning to clean it up when it has dried and produced a starch-like stiffness in the sheets. For personal reasons the young man does not want his mother (who presumably changes the sheets) to discover what has happened. The nocturnal emission, the wet-dream, is something to be ashamed of.

Where does this embarrassment about a perfectly natural phenomenon come from? Perhaps from the Bible. Leviticus 15:16–17, which is part of a code dealing with bodily emissions that render a person unclean, states: ''And if a man has an emission of semen, he shall wash his entire body in water and be unclean until evening. Every article of clothing and all skin which the semen contacts, must be washed and remain unclean until evening.'' It is not necessary to be aware of the specifics of the Levitical code for the influence of his ancient Hebraic attitude toward natural bodily functions to be felt; it has become a part of our environment as a sexual taboo.

The spontaneous nocturnal orgasm, which is also known as spermatorrhea, is not always associated with fantasy. Men with severed spinal cords, which destroyed the connection between the brain and the lower nerve centers, have experienced nocturnal emissions.[1] The orgasm can occur without the genitals being stimulated by hand or being rubbed against the night clothes, although some women have awakened to find their hand on their vulva, and some men have discovered that they have been in direct contact with the bed covers. On the other hand, fantasies do occur; and the combination of taboos against lustful imagery and the uneasiness that results from contact with the semen can produce feelings of guilt and contamination.

Dreams and fantasy are part of the normal mental functionings of humans. Although it is possible that sexual thoughts that arise during the day may be related to nocturnal emissions, it is quite possible for the mind to develop imagery that fits what the body is experiencing. Nocturnal emissions occur with varying frequency among younger males, and reports suggest that the dreams can come more than once a week or once every few weeks for males who are not active sexually either through intercourse or masturbation. The feelings of guilt and uncleanness arise out of education, in particular, the education given by religious organizations. The Catholic church labeled nocturnal emissions "pollutio," and in some sex-books this natural bodily action is listed in the category of "nocturnal pollution." Martin Luther treated the wet dream as a sort of disease requiring the remedy of marriage. Some medical authorities treated the seminal emission on the same level as urinating in bed, or even vomiting. It is not surprising that a young man might experience shame and want to hide "the evidence" from his parents. Nor is it to be wondered at that young males and females feel they must have "done something wrong" or that there must be "something wrong" with them for this to happen. Their faith must be inadequate. They must be thinking "dirty thoughts." They are becoming so "obsessed with sex" that even in sleep the obsession manifests itself.

Modern physiology, modern sex-studies, and modern therapists tend to accept the orgasmic dream as something not under ordinary rational control, as a mental image that does not imply lust or lasciviousness, and as an occurrence that is perfectly normal in which the body (sometimes aided by the mind) relieves sexual tensions. It is a happening that is neither right nor wrong, evil nor good; it is simply natural.

NOTE

1. Clelland S. Ford and Frank A. Beach, "Self-stimulation," in *Human Autoerotic Practices*, ed. by Manfred F. DeMartino (New York, 1978), p. 209.

28

Voyeurism

Voyeurism is listed as a minor sexual deviation in which an individual has an urge to repeatedly look at unsuspecting people, most often strangers, who are in the act of disrobing, are naked, or are engaging in some form of sexual activity. The act is covert and has given rise to the term "peeping Tom," perhaps because the violators are most often males. The voyeur does not seek sexual activity with the person being watched, but enjoys a feeling of sexual excitement that may result in a masturbatory act. Voyeurism usually begins during adolescence and can continue throughout adult life.

There are those who would include in the definition of voyeurism the viewing of pornographic films or looking at the nude centerfolds in sex magazines. However, this kind of voyeurism (if it can be called that) involves looking at persons who are posing or acting for the purpose of being viewed. They cannot know exactly who is looking at their pictures, but they are (presumably) indifferent to the fact that they will be seen. The true voyeur may enjoy the awareness that those being observed would be angry or otherwise upset if they knew they were being watched; this is not the case with the viewer of pornographic literature or films.

There are only two reports of what may be viewed as voyeurism in the Bible. In the first, King David watched Bathsheba as she took her post-menstrual bath. (2 Sam. 11). The royal palace, like other homes, would have had a cloth-covered area with open sides constructed on the roof to provide protection from the sun's rays but openness to any prevailing breeze. David was enjoying an afternoon nap—a custom that is still fairly common in the Near East. As the day began to cool he moved to the low wall that edged the flat roof. Because the royal residence would have been built on higher ground than surrounding dwellings and would perhaps have been a two-story building, as opposed to the smaller one-story houses of his people, King David could look down on the neighboring dwellings.

In the ancient Near East, houses were crowded together along narrow streets. Some were constructed in an "L" shape with a wall enclosing the "L" forecourt represented by the open part of the "L." Others had an interior court. Bathsheba evidently believed she was well shielded from view. There can be little doubt that if she had been aware that she was being watched, she would have been dismayed. There is no condemnation of David's voyeurism.

The second example of voyeurism is found in the story of Susanna—a writing that is not accepted in the bibles of Jews and Protestants but is accepted by Roman Catholics and is included in Chapter 13 in the Catholic version of the Book of Daniel. It is generally dated in the first or second century B.C.E. and has been called a "detective story"[1] and "one of the finest short stories in the world's literature."[2]

Susanna was the beautiful young Jewish wife of Joakim, a wealthy man who opened his home and gardens for the meetings of the Jewish community. Among those who came were two lecherous elders who observed that Susanna used to walk in the gardens following the morning meetings. Each man would pretend to leave and would return to spy on Susanna. One day the two men came face to face, confessed their mutual desires, and planned to wait for an opportune time to entrap Susanna. On one particular hot day, Susanna, believing that all the guests had left, ordered the servants to close and lock the gates and to bring her bath equipment. When the olive oil and ointments had been brought, and the serving maids had left, the two elders came out of hiding and demanded that she yield to their sexual desires. When she refused, the elders opened the gates and called for the servants and charged Susanna with consorting with a lover who had fled.

The remainder of the story tells of Susanna's trial and sentencing on the basis of the accusations of the two witnesses, of Daniel's wise intervention as an attorney, of his questioning the two elders separately and uncovering the discrepancies in their stories and of the exoneration of Susanna. The story is one of a series of Daniel legends that were preserved and enshrined in the Vulgate Bible.

In actuality, the biblical accounts of David and Susanna differ from what is commonly called "voyeurism" today in that the voyeurs wanted to have sexual relations with the person being observed. They were not satisfied with observing. Their voyeurism had become lust and ended with attempts to have intercourse or, in David's case, actually having intercourse with the woman.

Voyeurism is condemned by Jews, Christians, and secularists. Not only is it a violation of an individual's privacy, but it can be a terrifying experience if the person being watched becomes aware of the voyeur. Because it is often a part of the maturation patterns in adolescence, it can be a source of guilt. Young children who do not have siblings of the opposite sex may take to a kind of curious voyeurism to see what the body of a person of the other sex is like. This often takes the form of peeking through bathroom or bedroom windows or peering through keyholes where the person watched is likely to have his or her genitals exposed. Most adolescents outgrow these inquiring peeping-Tom adventures. Those who do not pose problems in the communities where they live and often are apprehended by the law and referred for counseling to learn to cope with their asocial behavior.

NOTES

1. Bruce Metzger, introductory note ''Susanna'' in *The Oxford Annotated Bible with Apocrypha* (New York, 1965), p. 213.

2. Clyde M. Woods, introductory note ''Daniel and Susanna'' in *The New English Bible with Apocrypha: Oxford Study Edition* (New York, 1976), p. 188.

29

The Joy of Sex

Did the Hebrews not enjoy sex? Were there no moments of wild passion? No orgasmic explosions? No dazzling mental images of colored lights? Nothing of what someone has called the "Yah! Yah! Yah!" experience? Was sexual expression as rule-controlled as the Bible sometimes seems to make it?

The very fact that the Bible contains regulations to control sexual behavior indicates that what was forbidden and condemned was being practiced. There were whores and adulterers, transvestites and masturbators, and rapists and incestuous individuals. There were also lovers, and there was joy in sex. The one biblical book that gives testimony to the joy is the Song of Songs—a poetic work concerned with love and lovers.

The Song of Songs—the title means "the best of songs" or "the song above all songs"—is a collection or anthology of poems reflecting the intimate, sensuous, and passionate feelings of lovers. Despite the fact that it was at one time attributed to Solomon (and who should know more about sexual relationships than a king with seven hundred wives and three hundred concubines?), there is a lack of unity or structure that suggests the bringing together of independent poems. Moreover, the speakers—and the book is composed of monologues and choruses—are not identified and the geographic settings seem to vary. The book is a composite.

There are no theological themes. Indeed there is no mention of deity. No moral judgment is passed on sexual behavior. The Jewish leaders who accepted the book into the canon at the close of the first century of the Common Era allegorized the poems as expressions of Yahweh's divine love for his people Israel. Later, the Christian church dutifully followed the allegorizing interpretation and insisted that the poems were to be recognized as stating Christ's love for his church. Some modern scholars have found parallels in Syrian folk lyrics used in wedding ceremonies; others have argued that the poems were derived from ancient religious liturgies associated with dying and rising gods or with the fertility cult. Still others have attempted to analyze the dramatic structure of the collection, suggesting that it records a love affair between Solomon and a country girl. No matter which interpretation is accepted, the sensuous aspects of the poems are recognized. It is not impossible that the poems did originate in a non-Hebrew cultic setting as expressions of the love between deities, but they also reflect epithalamia in a peasant setting in which the language of love used by gods and goddesses in the cultus became or reflected the language used in wedding rites.

The poems express continuing delight in the form of beauty of the beloved and in touching, kissing, and making love. There is longing and desire present, as well as sexual imagery and erotic expressions, and they are stated by both partners. She is no passive partner and he is no macho lover! The ideals of beauty do not seem to have changed much over the centuries, but the love language of the Song of Songs reflects its several-thousand-year-old setting and employs descriptive terms that differ from what one might use today while making love. If the reader of the poems who knows and enjoys sex and love can move beyond the barriers of time, space, and verbiage and enter into the feelings of the poets, the passages are as sensuous today as they must have been in ancient Israel.

The opening words express desire:

> O kiss me with the kisses of your mouth
> For your love-making is better than wine,
> Your scented ointments are a delight,
> You are [smooth as] flowing oil.

[1:2 f.]

There is warm intimacy in the woman's expression of her feelings:

> To me, my beloved is like a cachet of myrrh
>   lying between my breasts.
> To me, my lover is like a cluster of henna
>   in the en-Gedi vineyards.

[1:13–14]

En-Gedi is a spring that gushes from the barren, golden, arid wasteland above the Dead Sea. Its waters flow to the sea, providing a lush, fernlike green gash between the flanking cliffs. It is not clear whether sexual body imagery was in the mind of the poet, but sensual imagery was certainly present.

The woman continues her ecstatic praise of her lover:

> He carried me into the wine house
> his banner [standard] over me is love.
> Sustain me with raisin-cakes, refresh me with apples,
> For I am weak with love.
> His left hand cradles my head
> His right hand embraces me.

[2:4–6]

Raisin-cakes were the sacred food associated with the fertility goddesses in ancient Canaan and Israel.

After the woman had retired to her home, she heard her lover at the door. He spoke:

> Open to me, my sister, my beloved, my dove, my pure one;
> For my head is wet with dew, my curls with the night-mist.

The woman noted:

> I had removed my garment, how could I put it on?
> I had washed my feet [sexual organs?] how could I soil them?
> My lover put his hand to the hole [in the door]
> And my heart longed for him [Literally: my bowels were moved for him—
>   the bowels were believed to be the seat of the emotions]
> I arose to open to my beloved
> And my hands dripped myrrh
>   my fingers liquid myrrh
> On the bolt of the door.
> I opened to my beloved
> But my lover had turned and gone.
> My spirit failed me when he spoke.
> I looked for him, but did not find him.
> I called to him and he did not respond.

[5:2–6]

Excitement, longing, desire, remorse, feelings of loss—all are expressed in these lines. She searched for him but could not find him. The watchmen who discovered her wandering about town at night beat her and took her cloak. She was, in her words, "sick with love" for her lover, who was described as being radiant and ruddy, with black wavy hair, dove's eyes, cheeks like a bed of spices, lips like myrrh-distilling lilies, a body like carved stone, and as tall and stately as a cedar of Lebanon. His words were sweet and he was absolutely desirable. He was both friend and lover [5:10–16].

The man too was overcome by love for his beautiful lover. His descriptive terms reflect the rural environment. Her eyes behind her veil are the soft eyes of a dove, her dark, rippling hair is like the movement of a flock of black goats down a mountainside, her perfect teeth are as white and even as freshly shorn and washed sheep, her lips are like a scarlet thread in her lovely mouth, her stately neck, with the encircling collar of row on row of coins, is like the shield of a warrior gracing David's tower. Her breasts are like two fawns. She is all love; she is perfect! Although the image of the movement of goats may seem strange to us, to anyone who has watched a large herd of goats come in waves down a Palestinian mountainside, the imagery for rippling black hair is beautiful. Bedouin women still wear chokers of coins that give the impression of stately necks.

The man, so completely overcome by his longing for the woman, attempted to describe his feelings. Her love is better than wine, her lips are nectar, her tongue and mouth like honey and milk, and her fragrance like an orchard of scented plants (4:10–15).

He begins to describe her again, this time from the feet up. Her feet in their sandals are graceful, the curve of her thighs like the work of a master craftsman, her round navel like a little bowl from which to drink wine, her abdomen like a mound of golden wheat with a border of lilies. Her breasts are like two fawns, her neck like an ivory tower, her nose like the crag overlooking Damascus, her head like Mount Carmel, and in her flowing tresses the lover is held captive. He returns to her breasts:

> Your very stature is like a palm tree and your breasts
>   its clusters
> I say, I will climb the palm tree and take hold of its
>   branches.
> Let your breasts be as clusters of the vine,
>   the scent of your breath like apples
> And your kisses like the finest wine that glides
>   smoothly over lips and teeth.

[7:1–9]

The woman could only declare: "I am my beloved's and his desire is for me" (4:10). She is no madonna on a pedestal, nor is she a whore. She represents a normal woman responding to her normal sexual feelings of desire for the man she loves.

The Song of Songs can be important in helping those raised in strict religious environments, which often tend to place negative emphases on human sexuality and sexual feelings, to discover that there is a biblical precedent for "letting go" in a sexual situation. The writing suggests that sex can be enjoyed in and for itself and that sex for pleasure was as important in biblical times as it is today. In other words, nice people, biblical people, also enjoyed sexual intercourse. Therapists often encounter situations in which couples experience various kinds of sexual problems because of rigid religious upbringing that has tended to make sex something that nice people do not do except to produce babies.

She is twenty-eight and her husband, who is a successful physician, is thirty-seven. He is the product of a home and church where fundamentalist biblical religion surrounded him from infancy. His family was not given to open physical expressions of love and caring. This couple has been married for three years and the young wife complains that she is not enjoying their sexual life because her husband will only respond to her when she dons miniskirts, black nylons with a garter-belt, a black lacy bra and panties, high heels, and make-up. She wants to be able to enjoy sex without "dressing up" in this special garb. She has tried soft feminine clothing, but if her husband does respond, he says, "No more." She says, "I feel like a whore."

Her husband has put her on a pedestal, where as his wife he feels she belongs. Only when he can perceive her as a "bad woman," which in his mind is identified with this particular costuming, can he bring himself to have intercourse with her. He believes that "nice girls don't," and he cannot bring himself to copulate with his wife, who is a "nice girl." He has to have her transform herself into his notion of a "hussy"—a bad girl—and with this other woman he can engage in sex. His religious education never put him in touch with the warm responses of the Song of Songs.

She is fifty-three and her husband is fifty-five. They have been married for thirty years, have raised a family, and have always enjoyed their sexual life—but he has always been the initiator. Now, because he is older, he feels the need for additional stimulation to bring him to erection and he has asked her to help him initiate sex. She responded: "I can't." What she really meant was "I am not willing," since there was no physical impediment. As their counselor, I suggested that, when they were in a "safe" place, in bed, she caress his body—not his genitals, just his body—his chest, shoulders, stomach, back. She protested: "I couldn't, I simply couldn't." Why not? Because her religious background had imprinted upon her that "nice girls don't"—they may be acted upon by their husbands, but they do not initiate sex or make open expressions of desire. Re-education was important. The Song of Songs helped her understand that in at least one book of the Bible "nice girls do" and that there is nothing "wrong" with letting the man know that she enjoyed and desired his loving attention and his body and that she was willing to cooperate in making the sexual experience happen.

One of the most positive contributions biblical literature can make to our present appreciation of human sexuality is the clear statement that sexual desire and the enjoyment of intercourse can continue into extreme old age. The implications of the statement that Moses was virile at the age of one hundred and twenty, and that Abraham continued to have an active sex life well beyond that age, has only started to permeate the thinking of those who deal with human sexuality among older persons with religious backgrounds. There is a popular folkloric notion that once a certain age is reached, interest in sex and the ability to perform sexually disappear. Recently, one young business executive lamented to his companions that now that he was thirty-nine he could only dread his forties—his wife would reach menopause and her sexual functioning would cease, and he would be too old to perform. One can only smile and contemplate the surprise that may be in store for him. But his thinking reflects the fact that he is absolutely out of touch with studies in aging and human sexuality. He is back with the undergraduates at Brandeis University, who in 1959 were asked to complete the sentence: "Sex for most old people . . ." Almost all added "unimportant" or "past" or "negligible" or similar descriptive terms suggesting that they believed that old people were "sexless."[1]

Studies by Masters and Johnson and other sex researchers have demonstrated over and over again how erroneous these ideas are and how injurious they can be if they are believed. They have found that older people can be sexually active and enjoy intercourse well into the eighties. The major problems encountered by these older men and women were the lack of a partner, which limited sexual activity to masturbation, and religious attitudes that suggested that sex for older people, and particularly sex for pleasure, was not proper. In addition, slogans like "dirty old man" and "dirty old woman" convey the message that there is something unclean or socially unacceptable about the elderly engaging in sex. As someone has said: What is virility at twenty-five becomes lechery at sixty-five. These negative attitudes reflect the mind-sets of those who, for religious or other reasons, are uneasy about human sexuality and sex.

The problem with these negative notions is that they just might be believed by the elderly man or woman. If the older individual is convinced that sexual impulses cease at a certain age or that sex involving an older man or woman is not quite nice, these beliefs can become the basis for self-fulfilling prophecies: believing that they should not be able to perform, they become impotent. Or they refrain from intercourse because they believe they should not engage in such activity. Repressed sexual feelings combined with the guilt the person experiences when these feelings continue can produce tensions.

Many elderly people decide to move to a retirement community or a rest home run by their church. One couple in such a home asked that the two single beds in their apartment be replaced by a double bed. They had slept together for more than fifty years of married life and were uncomfortable sleeping apart. The administrator, correctly discerning their desire for sexual intimacy, suggested that they were really too old for this sort of behavior. In another home, run by another denomination, a man of eighty and a woman of seventy-nine met, fell in love, and decided to get married and live together. They were discouraged by the administrator, who suggested that they were acting impulsively and that they needed more time—a year or two—to get to know one another better. The woman commented, "Who has time?" and the couple ignored the administrator's advice and were married immediately. Some religious organizations are out of touch with human sexuality.

In the section of this book dealing with May–December marriages, negative social attitudes were discussed. Often the raised eyebrows or the knowing leer reflects the notion that the older of the two will be an inadequate sex-partner. The woman was in her early twenties and the man she married was in his middle sixties. A former boyfriend and lover phoned her to wish her well.

During the conversation he asked, "But . . . do you do . . . everything?"

The bride smiled as she answered, "Everything!"

"But," the young man went on, "is he able . . . ?"

"Yes," came the answer, "and so much more beautifully and more often than anyone else."

Aging does bring physiological changes that affect sexuality. Menopause marks the end of potential child-bearing. For some women this event introduces a time of greater sexual enjoyment, freed of the fear of pregnancy or the need to use contraceptives. There may be some vaginal changes due to aging—greater difficulty in lubrication, a thinning of the vaginal walls, which by lessening the "cushioning" effect may make some positions for intercourse less comfortable, greater susceptibility to infection or inflammation triggered by estrogen deficiency, which in some cases may make intercourse difficult or painful. But despite these potential problems, sexual desire and capacity continue well into the eighties and even beyond.

As for the aging male, there is no physiological reason why sexual activity should not continue into the ninth and tenth decades of life. The arousal time is usually lengthened, sometimes the ejaculation is weaker and the seminal fluid is thinner, or the size of the testes may be reduced. These changes, if and when they occur, are minor and are parallel to other physical changes associated with aging. The biggest handicaps to sexual performance are the acceptance of folk tales pertaining to impotency and the lack of opportunity for sexual involvement. Sex counselors have found that fear of losing an erection or of not performing adequately are the most common contributors to male impotency—at any age. On the other hand, those males and females who remain sexually active throughout their lives appear to have few problems with sex in their older years. Nor is there any diminishing of enjoyment. As one male put it: "It may take a little longer, but it is just as good as ever!" His lover quoted her favorite paraphrase of an alcohol slogan: "Growing older is just getting better!" The young woman married to the older man said "No more frustration with males and their premature ejaculations. I can have several wonderful orgasms before my lover comes." These facts have given rise to a maxim that is popular in gerontological circles: "Use it or lose it!" The joy of sex is ageless.

NOTE

1. P. Golde and N. Kogan, "A Sentence Completion Procedure for Assessing Attitudes toward Older People," *Journal of Gerontology,* 14 (July, 1959), pp. 355–63.

Bibliography

Beyond the references listed in the footnotes, some of the following works have been useful resources. I have not included articles from the various religious encyclopedias that were also read, nor have I listed the biblical sources that include volumes from the International Critical Commentary Series, the Anchor Bible Series, the Cambridge Bible Series, the Interpreter's Bible, and the Interpreter's Dictionary of the Bible.

Acton, William, *Prostitution*. New York: Frederick A. Praeger, 1969.

Arnold, L. Eugene, ed., *Helping Parents Help Their Children*. New York: Brunner Matzel, 1978.

Barbach, Lonnie Garfield, *For Yourself: The Fulfillment of Sexuality*. New York: Doubleday, 1975.

Beach, Frank A., ed., *Human Sexuality in Four Perspectives*. Baltimore: Johns Hopkins University Press, 1976.

Bell, A. P., and Winberg, M. S., *Homosexualities: A Study of Diversity Among Men and Women*. New York: Simon & Schuster, 1978.

Berne, Eric, *Sex in Human Loving*. New York: Pocket Books, 1970.

Butler, Robert N., and Lewis, Myrna I., *Sex After Sixty: A Guide for Men and Women in Their Later Years*. New York: Harper & Row, 1976.

Cahnman, Werner J., ed., *Intermarriage and Jewish Life: A Symposium*. New York: Herzl Press and Jewish Reconstructionist Press, 1963.

Calderone, M. S., and Johnson, E. W., *The Family Book About Sexuality*. New York: Harper & Row, 1981.

Chesler, Phyllis, *About Men*. New York: Simon & Schuster, 1978.

Comfort, Alex, ed., *The Joy of Sex*. New York: Simon & Schuster, 1972.

Crooks, R., and Baur, K., *Our Sexuality*. Menlo Park, Calif.: Benjamin-Commings Publ. Co., 1980.

Dalton, Katharina, *Once a Month*. Pomona, Calif.: Hunter House, 1979.

Delaney, Janice, Lupton, Mary Jane, and Toth, Emily, *The Curse: A Cultural History of Menstruation*. New York: E.P. Dutton, 1976.

De Martino, Manfred F., ed., *Human Autoerotic Practices*. New York: Human Sciences Press, 1979.

de Riencourt, Amaury, *Sex and Power in History*. New York: Dell, 1974.

Diamond, M., and Karlen, A., *Sexual Decisions*. Boston: Little, Brown, 1980.

Edwardes, Allen, *Erotica Judaica*. New York: Julian Press, 1967.

Ellis, Albert, *Sex Without Guilt*. New York: Lyle Stuart, 1958.

Ellis, John Tracy, *American Catholicism*, 2nd ed. Chicago: University of Chicago Press, 1969.

Ellis, Havelock, *Psychology of Sex*. New York: Emerson Books, 1933.

Fischer, Joel, and Gochros, Harvey L., eds., *Handbook of Behavior Therapy with Sexual Problems* (2 vols.). New York: Pergamon Press, 1977.

Fisher, Seymour, *The Female Orgasm*. New York: Basic Books, 1973.

Forward, Susan, and Buck, Craig, *Betrayal of Innocence: Incest and Its Devastation*. Baltimore: Penguin Books, 1979.

Gagnon, J., and Simon, W., *Sexual Conduct: The Social Sources of Human Sexuality*. Chicago: Aldine, 1973.

Goldberg, B. Z., *The Sacred Fire*. New York: Horace Liveright, 1932.

Goldberg, Herb, *The Hazards of Being Male*. New York: Signet Books, 1976.

Gordon, Chad, and Johnson, Gayle, eds., *Readings in Human Sexuality: Contemporary Perspectives*. New York: Harper & Row, 1976.

Green, R., ed., *Human Sexuality: A Health Practitioner's Text*. Baltimore: Williams and Wilkins, 1975.

Green, Richard, *Sexual Conflict in Children and Adults*. Baltimore: Penguin Books, 1974.

Hite, S., *The Hite Report: A Nationwide Survey of Female Sexuality*. New York: Macmillan, 1976.

———, *The Hite Report on Male Sexuality*. New York: Alfred A. Knopf, 1981.

Holt, John, *How Children Fail*. New York: Dell, 1964.

Hughes, Philip, *A Popular History of the Catholic Church*. New York: Macmillan, 1947.

Hutchison, J. B., ed., *Biological Determinants of Sexual Behavior*. New York: John Wiley and Sons, 1978.

Jersild, Paul T., and Johnson, Dale A., eds., *Moral Issues and Christian Response*. New York: Holt, Rinehart and Winston, 1971.

Kahn, Sandra S., and Davis, Jean, *The Kahn Report on Sexual Preferences*. New York: Avon Books, 1982.

Kaplan, Helen Singer, *Disorders of Sexual Desire*. New York: Brunner Matzel, 1979.

———, *The New Sex Therapy*. New York: Brunner Matzel, 1974.

Katchadourian, H., *Human Sexuality: Sense and Nonsense*. W. H. Freeman, 1972.

Katchadourian, Herant A., and Lunde, Donald T., *Biological Aspects of Human Sexuality*. New York: Holt, Rinehart and Winston, 1972.

Kriegal, Leonard, ed., *The Myth of American Manhood*. New York: Dell, 1978.

Lynd, Helen Merrell, *On Shame and the Search for Identity*. New York: John Wiley and Sons, 1967.

Maisch, Herbert, *Incest*. New York: Stein and Day, 1972.

Malfetti, James L., and Eidlitz, Elizabeth M., eds., *Perspectives on Sexuality*. New York: Holt, Rinehart and Winston, 1972.

Marcus, J. M., and Francis, J. J., eds., *Masturbation from Infancy to Senescence*. New York: International Universities Press, 1975.

Masters, R. E. L., *Sex-Driven People*. Los Angeles: Sherbourne Press, 1966.

———, ed., *Sexual Self-Stimulation*. Los Angeles: Sherbourne Press, 1967.

Masters, William H., and Johnson, Virginia E., *Human Sexual Inadequacy*. Boston: Little, Brown, 1970.

———, *Human Sexual Response*. Boston: Little, Brown, 1966.

Mitchell, Roger S., *The Homosexual and the Law*. New York: Arco, 1969.

Montagu, Ashley, *Sex, Man and Society*. New York: G. P. Putnam's Sons, 1963.

O'Dea, Thomas F., *The Mormons*. Chicago: University of Chicago Press, 1957.

Ollendorff, Robert, *The Juvenile Homosexual Experience and Its Effect on Adult Sexuality*. New York: Julian Press, 1966.

Ostow, Mortimer, ed., *Sexual Deviation*. New York: Quadrangle, 1974.

Parker, Tony, ed., *The Twisting Lane: The Hidden World of Sex Offenders*. New York: Harper & Row, 1969.

Pleck, Elizabeth H., and Joseph H., eds., *The American Man*. Englewood Cliffs, N.J.: Prentice-Hall, 1980.

Pleck, Joseph H., and Sawyer, Jack, eds., *Men and Masculinity*. Englewood Cliffs, N.J.: Prentice-Hall, 1974.

Porteus, Hedy, *Sex and Identity: Your Child's Sexuality*. New York: Bobbs-Merrill, 1972.

Reik, Theodor, *Of Love and Lust*. New York: Farrar, Straus, 1949.

Reuther, Rosemary R., ed., *Religion and Sexism*. New York: Simon & Schuster, 1974.

Saddock, Benjamin J., Kaplan, Harold I., and Freedman, Alfred M., eds., *The Sexual Experience*. Baltimore: Williams and Wilkins, 1976.

Seaman, B., and Seaman, G., *Woman and the Crisis in Sex Hormones*. New York: Bantam, 1978.

Simons, Joseph, and Reidy, Jeanne, *The Risk of Loving*. New York: Seabury Press, 1973.

Sisley, Emily, and Harris, Bertha, *The Joy of Lesbian Sex*. New York: Simon & Schuster, 1977.

Socarides, Charles W. *Homosexuality*. New York: Jason Aronson, 1978.

————, *The Overt Homosexual*. New York: Grune and Stratton, 1968.

Sperry, Willard L., *Religion in America*. Boston: Beacon Press, 1963.

Stein, Robert, *Incest and Human Love*. Baltimore: Penguin Books, 1974.

Stekel, Wilhelm, *Impotence in the Male* (2 vols.). New York: Liveright, 1959.

Szasz, Thomas, *Sex by Prescription*. Baltimore: Penguin Books, 1980.

Van Doornik, N. G. M., Jelsma, S., and Van de Lisdonk, A., *A Handbook of the Catholic Faith*. New York: Doubleday, 1954.

Whitely, C. H., and Whitely, Winifred, *Sex and Morals*. New York: Basic Books, 1967.

Wolman, B. B., and Money, J., eds., *Handbook of Human Sexuality*. Englewood Cliffs, N.J.: Prentice-Hall, 1980.

Zilberberg, Bernie, *Male Sexuality: A Guide to Sexual Fulfillment*. Boston: Little, Brown, 1978.